THE BLACK HEALTH LIBRARY GUIDE TO DIABETES

Lester Henry, M.D.

with Kirk A. Johnson

Edited by Linda Villarosa
Health Editor, *Essence* Magazine

Nutritional Advisor, Maudene Nelson

Illustrated by Marcelo Oliver

HENRY HOLT AND COMPANY
NEW YORK

To all African-Americans who have suffered for lack of reliable information about diabetes.

Henry Holt and Company, Inc.
Publishers since 1866
115 West 18th Street
New York, New York 10011

Henry Holt® is a registered trademark of Henry Holt and Company, Inc.

This book is not intended as a substitute for medical advice of physicians and should be used only in conjunction with the advice of your personal doctor. The reader should regularly consult a physician in matters relating to his or her health and particularly with respect to any symptoms that may require diagnosis or medical attention.

Library of Congress Cataloging-in-Publication Data
Henry, Walter Lester.
   The Black health library guide to diabetes / Walter Lester Henry ; with Kirk A. Johnson ; edited by Linda Villarosa. — 1st ed.
       p.   cm. — (The Black Health Library)
       "An Owl Book"
   Includes index.
       1. Diabetes.   2. Afro-Americans—Health and hygiene.   I. Johnson, Kirk A. II. Villarosa, Linda.   III. Title.   IV. Series.
   RC660.H46   1993   93–7152
   616.4′62′08996073—dc20   CIP

ISBN 0-8050-2285-6
ISBN 0-8050-2286-4 (An Owl Book: pbk.)

First Edition—1993

Designed by Kate Thompson
Produced by 2M Communications, Ltd.

Printed in the United States of America
All first editions are printed on acid-free paper. ∞

10 9 8 7 6 5 4 3 2 1
10 9 8 7 6 5 4 3 2 1   (pbk.)

THE BLACK HEALTH
LIBRARY GUIDE TO
DIABETES

Other titles in the Black Health Library:

Guide to Stroke
Guide to Heart Disease and Hypertension
Guide to Obesity

CONTENTS

FOREWORD

We call it "sugar," but it's hardly a treat.

One in ten black Americans—three million in all—have diabetes, and half don't even realize it. We are 55 percent more likely than whites to have diabetes, substantially less likely to have access to high-quality medical care, and much more likely to suffer the disease's crippling complications—dimmed eyesight, failing kidneys, amputated toes and legs. Diabetes is so common that some black families accept it as an inevitable part of aging. As one black woman confided in Pennsylvania State College of Medicine researcher Dr. Shiriki Kumanyika, "My family has diabetes so bad that people say you're not a member of the family unless your toes fall off when you get older."

Yet diabetes is anything but inevitable. In fact, one hundred years ago, diabetes in African-Americans was extremely rare. Only in the past few generations has the incidence of diabetes risen dramatically in the black community.

Historically, we have had precious few resources to counter this disturbing trend. For years there has been a desperate need for a comprehensive manual that everyone, even a person with no technical background, will find useful and reassuring.

A guide that explains what diabetes is, why black people are at risk—and more important, what we can do to minimize that risk.

A tool that helps diabetics and their friends and families successfully engage the challenges of diabetes.

A compilation of the latest medical developments and the most farsighted recommendations tailored expressly to the black community.

A user-friendly guide dispensing straight talk, comforting words, and hope.

This is such a book.

Chapter 1 ("What Is Diabetes?") opens with an easy-to-understand explanation of what diabetes is, what causes it, and how prevalent it is among black Americans.

Chapter 2 ("What Does Diabetes Do?") explains the diverse

health complications that diabetes can cause, particularly in African-Americans, and why diabetes deserves our respect.

Chapter 3 ("Black Folks at Risk") explores why African-Americans have more diabetes than other communities and answers the question that some may be afraid to ask: "Are black folks inherently prone to diabetes?"

Chapter 4 ("So You've Got 'Sugar'") explains what the symptoms of diabetes are, how doctors diagnose the disease, how a doctor should examine you, and what doctors prescribe for diabetics.

Chapter 5 ("Living with Diabetes") discusses how to cope with the emotional impact of the disease, plus helpful "do's and don't's" for diabetics.

Chapter 6 ("Watching What You Eat") explains why a good diet is all-important for diabetics and introduces time-tested ways to stay on track.

Chapter 7 ("Exercising Your Options") tells why doctors recommend exercise for diabetics, and explains how how you can actually make exercise fun.

Chapter 8 ("Taking Your Medicine") covers the ins and outs of insulin and diabetes pills—what they're called, how they work, when they should and shouldn't be prescribed, and which medicines are most useful for African-Americans.

Chapter 9 ("Helping Our Most Vulnerable") discusses children, pregnant women, and the elderly—three sectors of our community at particular risk from diabetes—and what they and loved ones can do to protect against the disease.

Chapter 10 ("New Hope for Better Lives") lays out the promise of the future. It explains how new research will make life easier and happier for diabetics and what it will take to put an end to diabetes in the African-American community.

The book concludes with a list of resources, including how to get free medication, free referrals to diabetes experts, and free information about diabetes.

Please remember that no book can substitute for a health professional. Anyone who has diabetes or who recognizes possible warning symptoms should seek the care and advice of a physician or other professional. Use this book as a supplement to medical care, not a replacement.

We are indebted to the staffs of the Meharry Medical College Library and the Vanderbilt University Medical Center Library for their patient assistance in preparing this book. We also acknowledge the work of Martha Robinson, who labored hard to prepare a first draft of the manuscript.

L.H.
Washington, DC
K.A.J.
Nashville, TN
May 1993

WHAT IS DIABETES?

Thirty-five hundred years ago, somewhere in the fertile northeast tip of Africa, someone decided to compile a written record of what the ancient Egyptians knew about medicine. At the time, Egypt's prowess in anatomy and surgery rivaled its legendary advances in engineering, mathematics, and astronomy, and the scribe must have sensed the importance of preserving this precious knowledge. But as he put pen to papyrus, little did he know that he was recording the very first account of diabetes. One thousand years before the birth of Hippocrates—the man widely but perhaps incorrectly considered the "Father of Medicine"—a brown-skinned scribe was the first to tell the world about a bizarre disease that caused "the passing of too much urine."

Is it surprising that the first written account of a disease that affects so many African-Americans came from ancient Africa?

For thousands of years, men and women of all colors have tried to unravel the secrets of a baffling affliction that has puzzled doctors and patients alike. Early on, observers noticed that diabetics were ravenously hungry. They would eat huge portions of food but still lose weight. And diabetics were gripped by spectacular thirst—"thirst, as if scorched up by fire," wrote one early observer.

1

Yet no amount of water could satisfy them. As patients dwindled to skin and bones, they released prodigious amounts of urine. Thus Aretaeus, a renowned Greek physician, described diabetes as "a melting down of the flesh and limbs into urine. The patients never stop making water, but the flow is incessant, as if from the opening of aqueducts." It was Aretaeus who coined the word *diabetes* from the Greek word meaning siphon.

The other unusual thing about diabetics' urine, aside from its remarkable quantity, was its sweetness, an observation noted by scholars in India and China as early as 300 A.D. "The urine was wonderfully sweet," wrote one seventeenth-century physician, "as if saturated with honey or sugar." And so the word *mellitus* (meaning honey) was added to the name of this mysterious disease.

Then in 1889 a Russian scientist named Oskar Minkowski had a most fortunate argument with his colleague, J. von Mering. The disagreement was over whether a dog could survive without a pancreas. To settle the dispute, Minkowski removed the animal's organ. Lo and behold, the dog began to urinate profusely, and flies clustered around the sweet-tasting urine. Working with more dogs, von Mering and Minkowski were amazed at how removing the pancreas made formerly contented animals nervous and anxious. "With extraordinary greediness, they threw themselves at any time upon the food which was offered to them," the scientists wrote, "even when they had, only a short time before, been amply fed, and all the time they looked around for every drop of water they could get hold of." Only one conclusion made sense: "After removal of the organ the dogs became diabetic."

Shortly thereafter, an American pathologist studying a young girl who had died of diabetes noticed deterioration of small clusters of cells scattered throughout the pancreas. These clusters, resembling tiny islets, had been first discovered by Paul Langerhans, a German pathologist. In 1916 a British scientist wondered if the islets of Langerhans, as they were called, might produce a substance that affects how the body burns carbohydrates. He named this theoretical substance *insulin*.

Then came the medical discovery that rocked the world. In 1921, a Canadian surgeon by the name of Frederick Banting teamed up with an enthusiastic graduate student, Charles Best, to crack the insulin riddle. Working with virtually no money in a laboratory borrowed from a vacationing professor, Banting and Best painstakingly prepared insulin-containing extracts from the islets of Langerhans and injected them into a sickly dog that had been made surgically diabetic. Within two hours the dog's condition began to improve and the amount of sugar in its urine started to fall. The dog eventually made a complete recovery. That, then, was the key! Diabetics became sick because their pancreas didn't secrete enough insulin.

Banting and Best tested their theory by giving insulin to a fourteen-year-old boy who was wasting away from diabetes. The child's recovery was near-miraculous. Before long other diabetic children had shown up at the pair's doorstep, some of them only weeks away from death. Insulin saved them all. A new era had dawned.

We've come a long way since the days of ancient Egypt. And although there's a fair amount about diabetes that we still don't understand, researchers know more than ever about what the disease is and what causes it.

DIABETES IN BRIEF

Diabetes is a disorder of metabolism—the process that supplies the body with energy. Like a cruising automobile needs a steady supply of gas, we need a constant supply of fuel to power our body's vast machinery. Climbing out of bed this morning, thinking about your day ahead, digesting your lunch, even taking a nap requires energy. We get the energy for these and a thousand other daily tasks—breathing, smiling, coughing, running, yawning, relaxing, dressing, scratching, speaking, dozing—from food.

A typical day's supply of food in America—perhaps cereal and fruit for breakfast, a sandwich for lunch, and meat and a few vegetables plus dessert for dinner—provides a mix of carbohydrates, proteins, fats, vitamins, and minerals. But when they pass through the digestive tract, many of the carbohydrates (starches and sugars) in this diverse collection of nutrients are broken down into what doctors and nutritionists call a simple sugar—glucose. Glucose is the body's principal fuel; it is to people what sunlight is to plants. The organ at the very center of the transformation of carbohydrates into energy-giving glucose is the pancreas.

The human pancreas is a curious organ (Figure 1). Shaped like your tongue and tucked away behind the stomach, this pinkish-yellow organ is inconspicuous. But without it, our bodies would slide into a metabolic tailspin. The pancreas secretes insulin, the hormone responsible for using and storing glucose.

Here's how the pancreas works. When you eat carbohydrate-

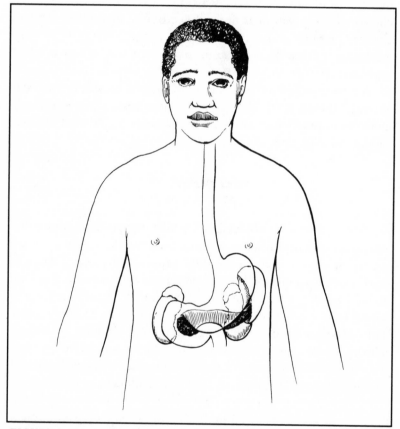

FIGURE 1 *The pancreas is a crucial player in carbohydrate digestion.*

rich food—a peanut butter and jelly sandwich, for example—the snack travels from your mouth to your stomach and on through the small intestine. Along the way, enzymes in your saliva and small intestine break down complex starches (in the bread) and sugars (in the jelly) into glucose, which passes through the lining of the small intestine and into the bloodstream.

Once it reaches the bloodstream, glucose is halfway home. But to get from the bloodstream to the individual cells throughout the body that need it, glucose needs a helping hand. That helper is insulin. In a healthy person, rising levels of glucose in the blood send a message to the pancreas gland. So-called beta cells in the islets of Langerhans start to secrete insulin, which pours into the bloodstream. Insulin finds the glucose and, like a mail carrier delivering a sack of letters, carries it from the bloodstream into millions of hungry cells from head to toe.

But that's only the beginning. When bloodstream insulin levels climb to a certain point, they send a message asking liver cells and fat cells to help handle the glucose load. The liver springs into action, storing excess sugar into a substance called *glycogen*. If you looked at a molecule of glycogen under a powerful microscope, you'd find several thousand molecules of glucose, all strung together in long branched chains. As for the fat cells, they do their part by using some of the extra glucose to manufacture more fat. (That's why people who eat too much food eventually put on weight.)

What happens between meals? When you go for a while without eating, your blood sugar level starts to fall. The amount of insulin in your bloodstream drops, too. (This protects against insulin reducing your blood glucose to dangerously low levels.) When the glucose level falls below a certain point, the pancreas is alerted once again. This time other cells in the islets of Langerhans start manufacturing a hormone called *glucagon*. Glucagon signals your liver to start breaking apart glycogen's long chains of glucose. Glucagon also teams up with cortisol, a hormone from your adrenal glands, which rest atop your kidneys. Together the two hormones manufacture glucose from body fat, or in extreme cases, from muscle protein. These safeguards help us maintain a normal level of blood sugar during sleep or fasting.

But occasionally these elegant checks and balances go awry. Sometimes pancreatic beta cells become destroyed, or there are too few of them to manufacture enough insulin to meet the body's demands. When this happens, the body can't deliver glucose into the cells. Sugar collects in the bloodstream, much like undelivered mail piles up during a postal strike. What's more, the low insulin levels trick the liver into thinking that the body needs fuel. In response, the liver breaks down glycogen and sends a stream of glucose into the bloodstream, where the sugar only adds to the high glucose levels already present.

In a panic, the body goes on red alert. The kidneys are mobilized to help flush huge amounts of excess sugar from the blood, thus yielding honey-sweet urine. Such large quantities of water are lost in the process that the diabetic becomes dehydrated and insatiably thirsty. At the same time, since there's no insulin to carry glucose into the body's cells, the cells literally starve despite being surrounded by food. In desperation, the body breaks down fat and muscle for nourishment, and the person loses weight despite eating everything in sight.

Meanwhile, the brain starts to reel. The breakdown of fat releases acids into the bloodstream, which begin to poison the brain. An important biochemical process involving phosphate, a vital mineral, goes haywire, causing brain tissue to lose its ability to take in oxygen. On top of it all, the relentless loss of urine dehydrates the brain. Without speedy medical attention, the brain eventually lapses into a coma. Death is near.

This is the classic and frightening picture of diabetes—the picture so graphically conveyed in historical accounts. More precisely, it's *Type 1 diabetes*, a form of the disease characterized by low or nonexistent insulin production. Type 1 diabetes used to be called juvenile-onset diabetes because it usually begins in adolescence or childhood. Scientists now know that this form of diabetes can affect persons of any age. Type 1 diabetics must receive insulin, usually more than once a day, to control their blood-sugar levels. This is why Type 1 diabetes is often called "insulin-dependent diabetes mellitus," or IDDM.

Like Type 1, *Type 2 diabetes* stems from an insulin disturbance. But in Type 2 huge insulin deficits aren't the problem. Type 2 diabetics usually manufacture enough insulin to sustain life. (That's why this form of the disorder is called "noninsulin-dependent diabetes mellitus," or NIDDM.) The problem is that the beta cells in the pancreas can't produce enough insulin to fully satisfy the body's needs. Under a microscope you can see why: the pancreas gland in Type 2 diabetics typically contains only half the normal amount of beta cells. Without enough insulin, glucose starts to accumulate in the bloodstream.

What's more, Type 2 diabetics are *resistant* to insulin. You may remember that insulin works closely with the liver. In a healthy person, the liver responds to high insulin levels by converting bloodstream glucose to glycogen for storage; low insulin levels trigger the liver to break down glycogen and send glucose back into the bloodstream. In Type 2 diabetes the liver doesn't respond to fluctuations in glucose levels. It releases a stream of glucose, regardless of the amount already circulating in the bloodstream.

In a healthy person, this so-called insulin resistance wouldn't be a problem; the body's various cells would simply take in the extra sugar and burn it as fuel. But in Type 2 diabetes, these cells are insulin-resistant, too. Cells are surrounded by a protective membrane; insulin normally works like a key that unlocks the membrane and allows cells to take in glucose. In Type 2 diabetes this lock and key no longer fit. It's like a mail carrier arriving at your doorstep only to find your mailbox welded shut. Instead, glucose destined for the cells winds up in the bloodstream where it joins the glucose that's already there because of inadequate insulin production.

Type 2 diabetes follows a different pathway than Type 1, but the result is the same: the fuel (glucose) that's so desperately needed to power every living cell winds up marooned in the bloodstream. This single metabolic error kicks off an extraordinary chain of events in the human body.

Doctors commonly divide the complications of diabetes into disorders that affect large blood vessels and those that affect small blood vessels. Among the large-vessel disorders are hardening and thickening of the body's principal arteries, which can lead to hypertension, heart attack, or stroke. When more distant arteries are involved, the result is circulation problems. For example, diabetics risk losing circulation and feeling in their limbs, particularly in their feet; diabetes is notorious for causing amputations of toes or entire legs.

Impairment of small blood vessels affects the eyes, causing slowly declining vision and even blindness. The kidneys are hit particularly hard; diabetes is one of the leading causes of kidney failure.

And there are miscellaneous disorders. Diabetes complicates pregnancies. It makes people's skin and muscles feel burned or prickly or numb. And it causes sexual frustration.

Indeed, one of the hallmarks of diabetes is just how extensive its reach is. "Heart disease is a one-organ disease," explained Dr. Donald Simonson of the world-famous Joslin Diabetes Center in Boston, in an interview with *Health* magazine. "But diabetes affects everything—biochemistry, physiology—everything."

WHO HAS DIABETES?

If diabetes were as rare as typhoid or the plague, we could at least take comfort that it touches few people. But this is an illness that afflicts over two hundred million people throughout the world, twelve million of them in the United States alone. The number of Americans with diabetes rose a surprising 17 percent from 1980 to 1987, and experts say the number will climb even higher. That's because the risk of developing diabetes increases as people grow older. And as the baby boom generation ages, the average age of our entire population creeps upward every year.

That's true for African-Americans, too. Black elders are growing faster in number than their white counterparts, and the future will surely bring more African-Americans with diabetes. Physicians say we don't have to wait to find rampant diabetes in our community: it's already here. African-Americans are just 12 percent of the population, but we comprise fully 20 percent of the patients diagnosed with diabetes, according to the National Center for Health Statistics. Diabetes is 16 percent more common among black men than white men, according to the National Diabetes Data Group, and 50 percent more common in black women than white women. Estimates vary, but up to one in ten black Americans has diabetes.

Most African-American diabetics have Type 2 diabetes; their pancreas produces some insulin but their bodies don't respond very well to it. Only a small number of African-American diabetics— perhaps 5 percent—have Type 1 diabetes. In fact, the incidence of Type 1 diabetes among blacks is only half that among whites. Because most black diabetics have Type 2 diabetes and usually don't need insulin, many take the disease for granted. In the face of urgent daily affairs—safeguarding our children, handling an obstinate landlord, caring for an elderly relative, fighting to improve our neighborhood schools, and squeezing in time for church, all while somehow managing to shop, cook, and earn a living wage—it's easy to sweep Type 2 diabetes under the rug.

In fact, for years many doctors felt that Type 2 wasn't very serious either, and they advised their patients not to worry about it. Not any more. Today, every black doctor recognizes that diabetes in either form cuts a terrible swath through the black community, leaving in its wake broken bodies and heavy hearts. Diabetes kills one thousand Americans every day, and a disproportionate number are African-Americans. Physicians and researchers have labored for many years to uncover the secrets of diabetes, and the most logical place to start is by asking what causes this mysterious affliction. Here are the most likely answers.

WHAT CAUSES DIABETES?

If you're like most people, chances are that when you catch a cold, you recover from it within five to seven days. Over the course of that week, your immune system recognizes an alien in your system—the cold virus—and sets about attacking and destroying it. In Type 1 diabetes, the immune system leaps into action just as it does when it senses a cold coming on. But it makes a tragic mistake: instead of attacking foreign invaders, it goes after the pancreas, destroying the very beta cells that the body relies on to manufacture insulin.

After years of speculation, researchers think that Type 1 diabetes is an *autoimmune disease*, an affliction in which the immune system somehow crosses its wires and attacks the very body it was designed to protect. Several leading theories explain how such a nightmarish chain of events comes about. Some scientists say the problem lies with the immune system's scavenger cells. These *macrophages*, as they're called, function as scouts, drifting through the bloodstream in search of foreign matter or damaged cells. When they find it, they grind it up and insert fragments of chewed up protein into special grooves on the macrophage's spherical surface. That's the signal for T-cells, the body's exterminators. When circulating T-cells come along, they "read" the protein bits stuck to the backs of the macrophage cells. Then they rush off on a search-and-destroy mission, looking for anything that matches the protein they have just read.

Built into the system is an important safeguard. If a macrophage grinds up a damaged cell from a person's own body—for instance, a pancreatic beta cell that's been damaged by a virus—T-cells normally recognize that the protein fragments are from the person's own body. The immune system isn't activated. But in people prone to diabetes, the grooves on the back of the macrophage latch onto bits of ground-up protein that T-cells don't recognize as coming from the person's body. Instead, the T-cells assume their marching orders are to destroy more of the same. And that means killing healthy pancreas cells. It takes a number of years for the body's defenses to accomplish their errant mission, but they eventually do. Once a critical mass of beta cells no longer produces insulin, the result is diabetes.

Type 1 diabetes is thought to stem from other factors as well. When we receive a transplanted organ, the natural tendency of our bodies is to reject the foreign tissue. That happens because of so-called Human Leucocyte Antigens, or HLA. (An *antigen* is foreign matter that the body attacks with destroyer cells called antibodies.) Researchers have characterized these antigens in great but not complete detail. Suffice it to say that the fifty-seventh amino acid on a certain chain of a certain HLA helps determine a person's resistance or susceptibility to Type 1 diabetes.

Genetics plays a role, too. If one identical twin has Type 1 diabetes, there's a 25 percent chance that the other twin will have the disease as well.

Not everyone agrees on how Type 1 diabetes starts, but most accept the idea that for one reason or another the body turns against itself. Type 2 diabetes, on the other hand, is usually caused by something entirely different: too much body weight. Eighty percent of American Type 2 diabetics are obese. For reasons not yet clear, excess body weight renders cells resistant to insulin. Even in healthy people, obesity makes the body's cells less responsive to insulin than in people who weigh less. That causes sugar to accumulate in the bloodstream.

In response to too much bloodstream sugar, a large person who is healthy simply manufactures more insulin; hefty nondiabetics typically have two to three times more bloodstream insulin than do hefty diabetics. But some people simply can't produce the extra insulin the body needs. "These people can still make insulin, but they don't secrete it at the proper levels," Dr. Graeme Bell, a University of Chicago diabetes expert, explained to the *Chicago Tribune*. When this happens, bloodstream sugar levels climb ever higher, ironically boosted by glucose released from the liver. "By that time," says Bell, "the patient has diabetes."

The remarkable thing about Type 2 diabetes is that it appears to be largely preventable. Since the disease depends virtually entirely on body weight, people prone to Type 2 diabetes can often avoid it by watching their weight. We'll explore the important role of weight control in Chapter 5 and throughout the book.

In addition to obesity, Dr. Bell and others have arrived at a second explanation for noninsulin-dependent diabetes. They suspect that one reason Type 2 diabetics fail to produce enough insulin is a defective gene.

The scientists base their prediction on the careful work of Dr. Stefan Fajans of the University of Michigan, who spent thirty-two years studying a single French family. The family had an unusually high rate of Type 2 diabetes; of 275 family members in the study, over 40 were diabetic. When Dr. Fajans took a close look at genetic material from every family member, he found that those with diabetes appeared to have a different gene than the others. The gene controls an enzyme found in the beta cells of the pancreas gland, where it helps the beta cells sense the amount of glucose in the blood. If blood sugar levels rise, the enzyme normally signals the beta cells to secrete insulin. But if the gene responsible for creating the enzyme is faulty, the beta cell's sugar sensor might not function correctly. And that could be a reason why the pancreas fails to pump out enough insulin. "We've been looking for such a gene for a long time," announced Dr. Bell. "We think it's a smoking gun."

If an identical twin develops Type 2 diabetes, there's an almost 100 percent chance that the other twin will, too. Further research on the genetics of Type 2 diabetes could help reveal why.

Researchers throughout the world are closing in on what causes diabetes. That's an exciting prospect because it means tomorrow may bring a cure. Today, though, one thing is clear: whatever the origins of this disease, and by whatever mechanism it occurs, the effects of diabetes can be profound. Let's take a closer look at how diabetes affects African-Americans and what medical science can do to help.

WHAT DOES DIABETES DO?

The central dilemma in diabetes—not getting enough fuel to the body—is so fundamental to life that the disease causes widespread complications—"complications that ultimately encompass virtually every system of the body and every specialty of medicine," says Dr. Robert Ratner, Director of the Diabetes Center at the George Washington University Medical Center. "To know diabetes—it has been said—is to know medicine and health care."

If that's true, then the racial inequities that mark American health care should also be evident with diabetes. Listen to Dr. Michael Byrd, a African-American physician and medical historian at Meharry Medical College who has studied race and health care from antiquity to the present. "Black Americans are sicker than white Americans because of a health deficit that stretches back 370 years to slavery and beyond," Dr. Byrd lectures attentive black medical students throughout the country. "For a kaleidoscopic matrix of reasons, the slave health deficit has never been rectified."

That's certainly true with diabetes, a disease that can affect virtually anyone, but whose many complications rain disproportionately on African-Americans and other persons of color. To understand the impact of diabetes in our community, it's important to appreciate how diabetes affects our bodies and how it alters the normal workings of the cardiovascular system, the nervous system, and organs that are critically important for good health.

DIABETES AND THE CARDIOVASCULAR SYSTEM

Hypertension, Atherosclerosis, Heart Disease, and Stroke

Can you remember the last restaurant meal that you really enjoyed—an experience that you raved about to your friends or that you wanted to repeat? I'll bet you had great service: the waiter or waitress was attentive to your smallest need, bringing your meal exactly when you wanted it, refilling your glass as often as you needed, quietly whisking away your dishes as soon as you were through. Your waiter was your transportation system, delivering or disposing of whatever you needed to make your meal a success.

In a very basic sense, the cardiovascular system serves the same purpose. Through a vast and intricate network of arteries, veins, and capillaries, it delivers to each cell the oxygen, hormones, fuel (glucose), and various nutrients needed to grow and thrive. At the same time, it is a conduit for trash—carbon dioxide, damaged cells, waste material, and other disposables, which it carries to the lungs and kidneys for elimination. And it's all powered, of course, by the energetic pump that is our hearts. The heart circulates our blood from our arteries through our capillaries and back again via the veins—a roundtrip journey every drop of blood makes one thousand times a day.

At first glance, it may not seem obvious that something as seemingly innocent as sugar could damage your bloodstream. But it does. Thanks in part to excess sugar, diabetes contributes to such serious ailments as high blood pressure, poor circulation in the legs and feet, narrowing and hardening of the arteries, heart disease, and stroke. Diabetes has a particular effect on the body's smaller blood vessels, resulting in disorders of the eyes and kidneys.

How does extra blood sugar cause so much damage? Doctors aren't sure, but Dr. Michael Brownlee has one idea. Brownlee, a researcher at the Albert Einstein College of Medicine in New York City, says glucose likes to combine with other substances, like proteins. Excess glucose combines with proteins in the blood and in the walls of blood vessels to make sticky fragments that clump together in a sort of "biological superglue." Like a paper cut on your finger, this superglue is a constant irritation to the body, which unfortunately tries to repair the damage by growing new cells around it. In the bloodstream, these cells thicken the walls of arteries and capillaries.

Doesn't thicker simply mean stronger? If you're building a house, perhaps, but not if you're trying to keep your cardiovascular system healthy. The reason is that blood vessels need to stay supple and flexible. Your arteries—the vessels that carry blood away from your heart—are tubes of muscle cells surrounded by elastic fibers. This strength and elasticity make a perfect combination, because when your heart beats, the pulse of blood that surges through an artery makes the artery bulge. (During open heart surgery, you can actually watch blood ripple through the arteries with every heartbeat.) The elastic fibers help the arteries expand to accommodate each surge in blood. Immediately thereafter, the muscle tissue squeezes the artery, thus helping push the blood along to its destination. In this way, your arteries actually help your heart circulate your blood. Anything that thickens your arteries hurts their ability to expand and contract, and that means the heart has to work harder to pump your blood.

It also means narrower arteries, and that can bring on high blood pressure. To understand how blood pressure works, imagine connecting a revolving lawn sprinkler to a garden hose and turning on the water. The sprinkler would spin at a certain rate—say, fifty revolutions a minute. Now, if you replaced the hose with a narrower one and sent the same amount of water through it, the sprinkler would spin faster—perhaps one hundred revolutions a minute. That's because the pressure of the water is related to the width of the hose; the narrower the hose, the higher the water pressure. And that's exactly what happens inside the body. The narrower the blood vessels, the higher the blood pressure.

Blood pressure is also affected by your intake of fat and cholesterol. When we eat too much fat or cholesterol (sometimes called *lipids*), macrophages—the body's scavenger cells—incorporate some of the fat, thereby turning into a yellowish, waxy substance known as *plaque*. Plaque can bruise the inner lining of the arteries. Once it does, it opens a biochemical Pandora's box. Blood cells called platelets arrive on the scene, bonding with fatty plaque to form clots. Over time, these clots can grow so large that they narrow an artery substantially, or even block it. Narrowing the blood vessel contributes to hypertension, and more extensive blockage can cause a stroke if the clot cuts off the blood supply to the brain. It can also cause a heart attack if the blockage occurs in the blood vessels that supply the heart. Doctors call this lipid-induced narrowing and hardening of the arteries *atherosclerosis* (from *atheroma*, meaning fatty deposit, and *sclerosis*, meaning hardened).

Unfortunately, too much fat goes a long way. Early diabetes pioneer Dr. Elliott Joslin minced no words. "I believe the chief cause of premature development of atherosclerosis, save for old age, is an excess of fat, an excess of fat in the body (obesity), an excess of fat in the diet, and an excess of fat in the blood," wrote Dr. Joslin in 1927.

Indeed, the combined impact of hypertension and atherosclerosis is frequently devastating. Diabetics are twice as likely as others to suffer heart attacks or strokes. As dangerous as high blood pressure is in the general population, it's even risker for diabetics; one twenty-year study by the Equitable Life Insurance Company found that hypertension levels that were dangerous for otherwise healthy persons were downright perilous for diabetics.

For black diabetics, the picture is even more serious. Black and white diabetics appear to have comparable levels of bloodstream cholesterol, and black diabetics actually have a lower rate of heart attacks. But black diabetics have more hypertension than white diabetics do, just as black folks have higher rates of hypertension in the general population. As we've seen, this hypertension can lead to many of the health disorders that plague our community.

These are not merely occasional problems. About half of all Type 2 diabetics have high blood pressure at the time of diagnosis— a figure that soars to 70 percent five years after diagnosis. After fifteen years of diabetes, about 35 percent of all Type 1 diabetics have kidney disease, which is closely associated with hypertension.

Hypertension and atherosclerosis, diabetics' two most common problems involving the major blood vessels, are not inevitable. Hypertension can be successfully treated with several types of medication. *Diuretics* relieve the body of excess fluids; *beta blockers* make the heart pump less forcefully; *vasodilators* expand the arteries; *sympathetic inhibitors* dampen nerve impulses that would otherwise make the heart pump more blood.

Eating less sodium helps lower high blood pressure, too. Salt may make our food more appealing, but too much of it is dangerous to body tissues. When we eat too much sodium, our body dilutes the excess with water. As this salty water builds up in our blood vessels, it increases the pressure inside them, just like the pressure inside a tightly nozzled garden hose shoots up when you turn up the water.

Watching our diet can help reduce the risks of atherosclerosis as well as high blood pressure. You've no doubt heard doctors' advice to eat less cholesterol and less fat, especially saturated fat. These nutrients contribute to hardening and thickening of the arteries, as does cigarette smoking and obesity. If for some reason a good diet fails to lower the amount of fats in the blood, doctors can often do the trick with medication.

Eye Problems

Whereas damage to the large blood vessels affects the heart and arteries, damage to the fine blood vessels involves the eyes and the kidneys. In the eye, for example, diabetes causes a condition known as *retinopathy* (from *retina*, meaning eye, and *patho*, meaning disease). To understand why diabetics develop eye problems, picture driving a car into a bottleneck on a crowded city street. The street gets narrower and narrower, and as it does there's less space for everyone to fit on the road. Not wanting to hit your fellow drivers, you edge your car closer to the curb until finally you resort to an extreme: you drive onto the sidewalk and park until the traffic subsides. In essence, you've created your own impromptu thoroughfare.

With diabetes something similar happens inside the eye. Diabetes thickens the blood with glucose and extra clotting cells. It also thickens the membranes of the capillaries that blood must travel within the eye. The reduced blood flow stimulates the formation of new blood vessels—new thoroughfares for the blood—and connective tissue called *fibroblasts*. Unfortunately, these new capillaries are fragile and often bleed. And the fibroblasts—the connective tissue—become scar tissue. The combination of leaky capillaries and fibrous scar tissue can be ominous for the retina, the capillary-rich membrane that collects visual images for the brain. In fact, if fluid and scar tissue build up beneath the retina, the retina can actually detach from the tissue beneath it, causing serious vision problems.

Diabetes also heightens the risk of cataracts (which make the normally clear lens cloudy) and doubles the risk of glaucoma (buildup of pressure inside the eye). Together, these three conditions can cause everything from mild and reversible vision loss to severe blindness. In fact, diabetic retinopathy is one of the leading causes of blindness in the United States (Figure 2).

Sadly, blindness from diabetic eye disease is more common in blacks than in whites. That's partly because our community has higher rates of hypertension, which increases the risk of eye damage. But it's also because we don't seek medical care early enough. Experts say the best way to prevent eye damage from diabetic retinopathy is to make regular visits to an ophthalmologist, starting soon after you are diagnosed with diabetes. That way the eye doctor can examine your eyes before any symptoms develop, and you can get advice as soon as any complications begin. But black diabetics see eye doctors much too late in the game, according to a 1991 study at the King/Drew Medical Center in Los Angeles. Researchers there found that by the time black diabetics visited an eye clinic for help, 37 percent of them already had severe

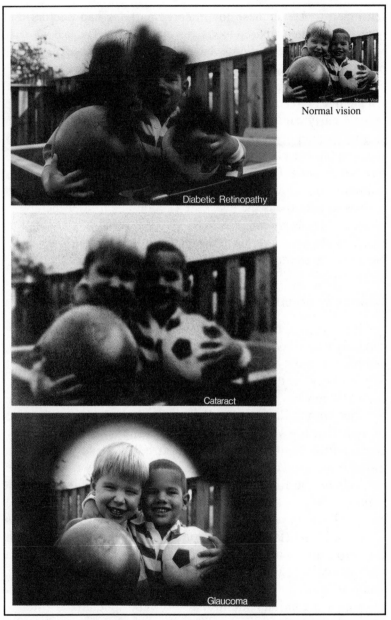

Normal vision

Diabetic Retinopathy

Cataract

Glaucoma

FIGURE 2 *The three eye disorders caused by diabetes: diabetic retinopathy, cataracts, and glaucoma. (Courtesy of National Eye Institute)*

retinopathy. All of these low-income patients had doctors, but many hadn't been advised to visit an eye doctor. "The lack of early referral for these patients has to be a major concern," the researchers said.

There are several good treatments for diabetic eye disorders. All are most effective when used early on. Insulin therapy can help reverse early capillary damage from diabetic retinopathy; laser surgery can neither cure nor reverse retinopathy, but it can halt its progression. For glaucoma, medication and laser therapy are effective treatments. The only treatment for cataracts is surgically removing the clouded lens and using contact lenses or special glasses to help focus the eye. One caution about laser therapy in blacks: it tends to cause keloids. So if you have glaucoma or cataracts and you're prone to develop these thick scars, laser treatment may be a second-best choice.

Kidney Problems

Have you ever noticed how manufacturers like to boast how carefully they filter their products? People who design advertising campaigns know that Americans appreciate purity. But "cold-filtered beer" and "clean-filtered gasoline" are small potatoes compared to what goes on each and every day inside your kidneys.

The human kidney is a dark purplish organ about the size of your fist. It owes its color to its rich supply of blood; every twenty-four hours, the body's entire blood supply passes through the kidneys over five hundred times. As blood enters the kidney, the first stop on its journey is something called a *nephron*. Nephrons are the workhorses of the kidney. They're essentially long convoluted tubes that remove waste products from the blood (Figure 3). Blood enters a nephron under high pressure, and when it flows through capillary loops into a rounded collecting chamber, that same pressure forces water, glucose, salt, and various impurities and waste products through the capillary membrane—a very specialized filter—and into the collecting chamber. Once these wastes enter the chamber, they travel the length of the nephron. Along the way, some of the water is reabsorbed so we don't get dehydrated. Eventually this mixture of water and waste products leaves the kidney as urine.

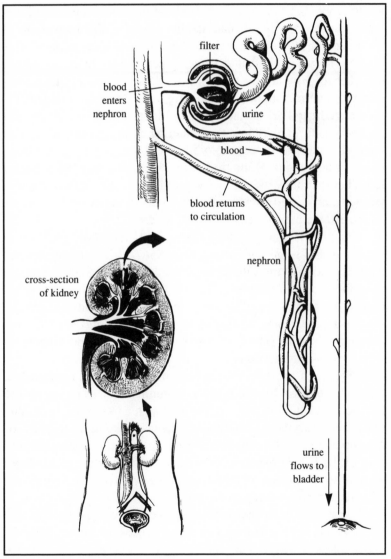

FIGURE 3 *Nephrons—workhorses of the kidney—filter blood to make urine.*

Each of our two kidneys contains around one million nephrons, and each nephron contains one filter. In diabetes something goes terribly wrong with this marvelous membrane: it begins to thicken. Over time it becomes less and less able to filter impurities and waste products from the blood. Without medical intervention, diabetics with kidney disease can literally drown in their own waste.

Researchers don't know for sure why diabetes causes this tragedy. They suspect that too much glucose in the blood stimulates the filter to grow until it becomes too thick to function. Hypertension plays an important role, too. High blood pressure hardens the specialized capillaries that filter the blood. As the capillaries get harder and stiffer, they lose their filtering ability. At the same time, diabetes forces the kidneys to work overtime to try to rid the body of too much sugar. Diabetic kidneys actually grow abnormally large because they are so overworked. Over the course of many years, what started as an exquisite filtering system simply shuts down, and the patient goes into renal failure.

Diabetes is the leading cause of an irreversible affliction known as *end-stage renal disease*, or *ESRD*, which often requires dialysis or kidney transplantation. Patients who get to this point are in serious condition indeed. "The medical, economic, and psychological impacts of this diagnosis are grave," concluded a team of Michigan researchers writing in the *American Journal of Kidney Diseases*, "and treatment is costly, cumbersome, and associated with serious complications."

ESRD is a growing problem in the United States, and it is a particular burden for the black community. For example, in the District of Columbia and surrounding states (Virginia, West Virginia, and Maryland), African-Americans make up 22 percent of the population. But in one recent year (1988), a whopping 56 percent of the ESRD patients were black. Nationwide, black people account for 31 percent of ESRD patients, over twice as high as our 12 percent representation in the general population.

Because the main causes of ESRD—diabetes, hypertension, and inflammation of the kidney's capillary loops—occur at an earlier age in blacks, ESRD occurs earlier as well. What happens when we develop kidney disease? Frankly, if we delay seeing a doctor or if we ignore the doctor's advice, prospects aren't very good. African-Americans recover from dialysis at a lower rate than whites do. One study of Michigan diabetics found that of over 7,400 diabetics and others with ESRD, only 211—not quite 3 percent—recovered sufficiently to leave dialysis. But black patients had a 38 percent lower chance of recovering from dialysis than did white patients.

The other treatment for ESRD—kidney transplantation—brings a different set of problems. Kidney transplants are now fairly routine operations, and diabetics who receive a kidney from a living related donor can look forward to an encouraging 80 to 90 percent survival rate in the first two years. The problem is that the demand for kidneys far exceeds supply, and African-Americans can't seem to get access to transplants.

Who receives kidneys and who doesn't was the question in a rather remarkable investigation by J. Michael Soucie of Atlanta's Emory University School of Medicine. After tallying over eight thousand ESRD patients in the Southeast, Soucie found that if you lived with a spouse and children and if you were employed, you stood a better than average chance of receiving a kidney. But if you had eight or fewer years of formal education, or medical complications such as visual impairment or cardiovascular disease, your chances were not very good. All in all, compared to white males, black males (whose risk of developing ESRD is *higher* than white males) had a 22 percent *lower* chance of receiving a kidney; black females (whose risk is even higher than black males) had a 34 percent lower chance. These statistics tell us that if you're black, if you're a single parent or gay or lesbian, if you're unemployed or never graduated from high school, or if you're sicker than others, chances are you'll still be standing in line while a white male rolls into the operating room to get his new lease on life.

On the whole, black people somehow manage to survive ESRD better than whites, despite our low survival rates on dialysis and our difficulty in receiving kidneys for transplants. But it is small consolation for the pain and risk of enduring such a difficult medical crisis. Small wonder that when doctors talk about the value of preventive care, ESRD is uppermost in their minds. Preventing ESRD is infinitely more effective than trying to cure it. "Diabetes and hypertension are treatable, and adequate control can prevent progression of renal failure," suggest Dr. Illuminado A. Cruz and colleagues at the Howard University College of Medicine. "However, with minority groups, it is difficult to fully implement the measures necessary to achieve this control." These and other researchers argue for wholesale education programs to help communities of color understand what we can do to prevent disease. "Ultimately," says the Howard University team, "these programs may be much cheaper than supporting a rapidly expanding ESRD program."

DIABETES AND NERVE PROBLEMS

Diabetics often suffer tremendous discomfort in their feet, legs, skin, and other parts of the body served by the so-called peripheral nervous system. That's been true for hundreds of years. Here's how one physician, writing in 1885, described his patients' distress:

> The usual account given by these patients of their condition is that they cannot feel properly in their legs, that their feet are numb, that their legs seem too heavy—as one patient expressed it, 'as if he had twenty pound weights on his legs, and a feeling as if his boots were a good deal too large for his feet.' Darting or 'lightening' pains are often complained of. Or there may be hyperesthesia [heightened sensations], so that a mere pinching up of the skin gives rise to great pain; or, it might be, the patient is unable to bear the contact of the seam of a dress against the skin on account of the suffering it causes.

Diabetes can still cause these nervous-system complications today. In fact, older diabetic amputees will often say that their problems started when they didn't realize that their numb feet were infected. The big difference is that today's patients have at their disposal a range of effective therapies to help relieve the painful symptoms and in some cases even prevent them from occurring.

If the cardiovascular system is our body's transportation network, the nervous system is our communication network. Nerves extend into every byway and crevice of our bodies, where they use electrical signals to relay commands from the brain (and sometimes the spinal cord) and return information about our environment to the brain. We rely on our nervous system more than you might think. As you read this paragraph, is the room chilly? Is the light adequate? Can you hear a clock ticking? Are you holding the pages in place with your thumb? Are you getting a little hungry? Is your mind drifting back to kidney transplants? Within us and around us lies a whirlwind of motion, sensation, memories. The fact that we can stand in the center of it all, taking in information and dictating our actions and responses, is a tribute to the marvelous internal circuitry that forms the brain and our many nerves.

Some patients wonder how to visualize a nervous system that they cannot see. I like to think of our nerves as shiny new telephone wires strung across the countryside, with our brain a command post instantaneously relaying and receiving thousands of messages each second.

With diabetes this glistening circuitry can begin to rust. Why? You may recall that diabetes is often accompanied by hypertension and atherosclerosis. These conditions affect nerves in a number of ways. Blood vessels that supply the nerves in the legs, feet, and skin can become blocked—sometimes completely—by fatty plaque, which is partly why diabetics experience such debilitating pain and numbness. If diabetes involves nerves that feed the gastrointestinal tract, you may have trouble digesting your food because the nerve signals that prompt muscles to push food through the system are misfiring. Food can get stuck in the throat because the esophagus no longer pushes each mouthful down to your stomach; your stomach can take a long time to empty; your gallbladder may not supply digestive enzymes properly; you can get diarrhea or constipation.

There's more. Diabetics often feel lightheaded when they stand up. That's because the muscles that normally compensate for gravity by pushing blood up into your head aren't receiving the proper nerve instructions. Profuse sweating is not uncommon in diabetes; it's a sign that nerves that supply the skin's sweat glands are confused.

You can see that our nerves are involved in many of the everyday activities we take for granted. When they start to misfunction, the resulting problems can affect much of our lives, including our intimate lives.

Sexual Disorders

Sexual problems are among the more debilitating frustrations of diabetes. Like all organs, the sexual organs are closely connected to the nervous system. Thanks to our nerves, our brain sends messages to our sexual organs (such as when we receive an arousing thought, sight, sound, or touch), and our organs transmit pleasurable sensations back to the brain. In men, control over erections resides in special nerve centers in the brain and spinal cord, and ejaculation occurs only because nerves signal certain pelvic muscles to fire. In women, lubrication of the vagina and the swelling of the labia and nipples during sexual arousal are all under nervous-system control.

It makes sense, then, that nerve damage from diabetes can seriously disrupt a person's sex life. For example, about half of all diabetic men complain that they have trouble achieving and maintaining an erection.

Some men also report poor bladder control. This, too, can affect sexual functioning. Urine and semen travel the same passageway, of course, and when a man normally ejaculates, the neck of the bladder is squeezed shut. Without this safeguard, semen can ejaculate into the bladder. This condition, known as retrograde ejaculation, happens in diabetics if the nerves controlling the neck of the bladder are affected by the disease. Fortunately, it is relatively rare, affecting only about two percent of male diabetics.

I should note here that sexual problems don't always stem from impaired nerves. A poor blood supply to the genitalia might be at fault; psychological factors can play a role, too. In some cases the side effects of medications prescribed for diabetes affect sexual functioning. These are discussed in Chapter 8.

Men who are struggling with these often difficult and embarrassing problems have several options. The Joslin Diabetes Center recommends first improving diabetes treatment, and discontinuing or changing any unnecessary medication. Next, it's often helpful to get back to basics, relearning sexual skills and rediscovering intimacy with your partner. This can start with an informal discussion with a doctor, or more formal counseling with a therapist. As a last resort, mechanical devices to help a man have an erection can be surgically implanted into the penis. At the Joslin Center, the satisfaction rate among men with implants runs as high as 80 to 90 percent.

Regrettably, sexual problems in female diabetics have been poorly studied. There is evidence, however, that diabetic women experience difficult arousal, painful intercourse, and a lack of orgasm. Changing medication may help if its side effects are at fault.

Nerve disorders are one of the many mysteries of diabetes, and there's a great deal that we don't yet know about them. We do know, however, that controlling your blood sugar can help relieve the discomfort of nerve damage. In fact, measures that reduce a diabetic's glucose intolerance can even *improve* nerve function. Remember: for people with Type 2 diabetes—and that includes most African-Americans who have the disease—reducing glucose intolerance means weight control.

A SPECIAL RISK OF DIABETES: INFECTION

Thanks to our immune system, our bloodstream is packed with an army of cells designed to protect us against bacteria, viruses, and other intruders. If you've ever seen a black diabetic who's missing a toe or worse, you may already know that diabetes can hurt the immune system; many cases of diabetic gangrene and amputation began with a blister, an ingrown toenail, or other infection so minor that a nondiabetic would scarcely give it much thought. Yet diabetics can and do suffer terrible infections of the skin, lungs (mostly tuberculosis and pneumonia), urinary tract, and even bone. Indeed, not too long ago, before the advent of antibiotics, infection was a leading cause of death in diabetes.

Dying from an ingrown toenail may sound farfetched, but it can happen if an infection isn't brought under control. Isn't that the point of the immune system? Well, yes, but diabetes weakens the body's infection-fighting cells, rendering them powerless to repel invaders. And that's not all. The body's first response to infection is to rush extra blood to the site to provide extra nutrients and infection-fighters for healing. But diabetics often have poor circulation, remember? As a result, sending first aid to the site of infection is like sending an ambulance down a dead-end road. Ironically, infection control is even more challenging because of the nerve problems associated with diabetes. As I mentioned, a numb foot won't even warn that you have an infection.

About 25 percent of diabetics eventually come down with infections and other problems involving their legs and feet. Perhaps one third of diabetics who have high blood sugar levels suffer from yeast infections of the skin. The risk of urinary tract infections is five times higher in diabetics than in nondiabetics. And there's a risk of gum infections, which can lead to gingivitis (gum inflammation), periodontal disease, and sometimes tooth loss.

These are just a few of the many infections that can make life very difficult for black and white diabetics alike. And yet black diabetics also face an extra risk of one of the saddest results of infection: amputation. On the whole, people with diabetes are fifteen times more likely than nondiabetics to lose a toe or leg to amputation. Black diabetics endure twice as many amputations as white diabetics do.

The happy news is that controlling diabetes also controls the risk of infection. If you manage the disease successfully, you shouldn't have to worry about the increased danger of foot infections, gum infections, and other similar problems. With today's knowledge of how to regulate blood sugar levels, say Drs. George Kozak and Leo Krall of the Joslin Center, "the susceptibility to infection has been largely overcome and approaches that of the nondiabetic." We'll examine how to guard against infection in Chapter 5.

- pregnancy
  complications
- what do I tell friends
  at meals
- alcohol/parties
  is it better to have
  hard liquor rather
  than beer
- letter for B.C.

384095

filofax

© 1994

February 1995

6 Monday

8:

9:

10:

11:

12:

1:

2:

3:

4:

5:

6:

7:

8:

FEBRUARY

M	T	W	T	F	S	S
		1	2	3	4	5
6	7	8	9	10	11	12
13	14	15	16	17	18	19
20	21	22	23	24	25	26
27	28					

PUTTING IT ALL TOGETHER

The preceding is but a small sampling of the many health risks that diabetes can bring. You can see why the disease has been so feared for thousands of years. Its reach is vast, and the complications are serious indeed.

But it's also important to realize that we've come a long, long way from the early days of diabetes, when "life is disgusting and painful," as one observer wrote, "and death speedy." Today, diabetes is anything but a death sentence. It's not a disease that we're powerless to stop. I see diabetes very differently than an affliction like lung cancer. If you have lung cancer, doctors can treat you with radiation or chemotherapy. You can also try any number of unconventional approaches, from a natural foods diet to meditation, which can't hurt. But the fact remains that even with the most vigorous therapy, the five-year survival rate for lung cancer is quite low. There simply doesn't seem to be very much that patients can do to alter the course of this terrible disease.

Diabetes is different. Over the course of my career, I have seen and treated thousands of African-American diabetics of all ages. I have watched patients grapple with the disease, and I have seen them come out on top. One of the most important lessons I've learned is this: *If you respect diabetes, you can survive it.* What many African-Americans fail to do is give the disease the respect it deserves. We take it for granted. We ignore warning signs. We fail to watch our blood sugar. We ignore our doctor's advice.

That's not respect. Respect is learning what we can about the disease. Respect is doing what it takes to stay healthy, and realizing that we can live life to the fullest but we have to take care of ourselves first. That respect—respect for ourselves, really—is important for all diabetics. But it's especially important for African-Americans, because the disease is so prominent in the black community. It occurs more often, it causes more severe side effects, and its consequences are more sobering.

Why does diabetes hit the black community so hard? Earlier in this chapter, I touched on some of the physiological reasons that black diabetics may be more prone than white diabetics to diabetes complications. But biological differences pale in comparison to some larger truths about black folks and diabetes—truths that just may surprise you. They all unfold in the next chapter.

BLACK FOLKS
AT RISK

Across the sunbaked sands of the Sahara desert travel a race of people whose day-to-day lives, like those of their ancestors, are relatively untouched by western influences. They are the Broayas, a small but unique tribe of nomads. Dark-skinned and straight-haired, they are blessed with extraordinary physical endurance and no obesity. They also have no diabetes.

Halfway across the world we find a very different scene. In the desert Southwest, the Pima Indians of Arizona have the highest rates of diabetes on earth. Here a staggering 40 percent of the males and over half of the females over age forty-five have diabetes.

Is diabetes a disease of race?

A casual observer might certainly think so. How else could you explain why the prevalence of diabetes differs so greatly from one race to another? How else could you make sense of the fact that Alaskan Eskimos have very low rates of diabetes, while Polynesians and Australian aborigines and African-Americans are practically overrun with the disease? In Type 2 diabetes—the type that most black diabetics have—we know the pancreas doesn't produce quite enough insulin. Could it be that the African-American pancreas simply doesn't function very well? Or maybe the problem is genetic. Remember the French study showing how Type 2 diabetics may have a defective gene? Could black people carry a gene that makes us susceptible to diabetes?

For some races, the evidence that diabetes runs along racial lines is undeniable. But that's not the case for African-Americans. If it were, black Africans would have the same high rates of diabetes that African-Americans have. In reality, Africans have relatively little diabetes.

Neither did African slaves. Medical accounts of slave health spoke of a number of diseases caused by poor nutrition or unsanitary living conditions. But nobody mentioned diabetes.

The fact of the matter is that diabetes wasn't a problem for African-Americans until sometime after the turn of the twentieth century. As the diseases of malnutrition and poor sanitation began to recede, thanks to better food and housing, diabetes began to emerge. When they appeared, the cases were alarming. A black physician wrote that one diabetic patient typically sat down to a breakfast of a dozen eggs, two pies, and a loaf of bread, and lost ten quarts of urine a day.

At first these and less severe cases of diabetes among black people were rare. In 1921 a physician writing in a black medical journal labeled diabetes a "perplexing condition that confronts the general practitioner from time to time." But by 1937, less than twenty years later, a doctor at Chicago's all-black Provident Hospital wrote, "It is the observation of many of the practitioners of our group that we are seeing an increasing number of cases of diabetes in our patients."

Half a century of health records from North Carolina show just how dramatically diabetes grew in the black community. In 1920 roughly 25 of every 100,000 elderly black people died of diabetes in North Carolina. By 1970 the death rate had soared to over 200 of every 100,000. Today, of course, the disease is rampant among African-Americans everywhere.

So something more than race must be at work here. As it turns out, the most important factor could be cultural: when rural cultures are westernized, the incidence of diabetes shoots sky-high. For example, in the southeast African nation of Tanzania, the diabetes rate among the rural Bantu tribe is among the lowest in the world—about 1 percent. But when rural Africans such as the Bantu move to the city, their lifestyle often changes radically. They give up their traditional diet of unrefined grains, starchy vegetables, wild greens, dried peas and beans, vegetables and fruits. Instead, they learn to enjoy western favorites—refined white bread, meats, sweets, alcohol. They become more sedentary, and they gain weight. All of these factors increase the risk of developing diabetes—so much so, in fact, that Africans who move to the city soon suffer diabetes rates as high as ours.

This is a worldwide phenomenon that's not confined to Africa. In the 1940s, for example, westernization hit Arizona's Pima Indians with a vengeance. In the 1940s, as they became acculturated to western living, the Pimas became more sedentary. They developed a yearning for hamburgers, white bread, instant pudding, and other fatty, sugary junk foods. And they became fat. These factors heightened their risk of diabetes. Whereas diabetes was once considered only a disease of industrialized nations, it is now spreading in epidemic proportions wherever native populations face encroaching westernization.

And so for our grandparents' parents, the act of being forcibly uprooted and thrust into the midst of a new culture, with new foods and new labor-saving machines, may have set the stage for a present-day diabetes epidemic that began to appear as black folks adopted more western ways.

You can see that lifestyle plays a significant role in whether or not someone develops diabetes. Lifestyle changes can even reverse diabetes once a person gets it. In Australia, to pick just one example, scientists have found that diabetic aborigines who return to their traditional diet and way of life show dramatic signs of disease reversal in as little as seven short weeks. This is an important point—and one I'll return to later— because too many of us assume that our health is largely a matter of fate or luck. It usually isn't. There is a tremendous amount that we can do both individually and as a community to be healthy.

Let's get down to specifics. Let's take a closer look at how the high rate of diabetes in our community is tied to our lifestyles—how we live, where we live, how we take care of our health. Along the way, we'll explore some of the reasons that certain African-Americans may be genetically prone to the disease.

OBESITY

When you find yourself putting on a few pounds, your partner may mention that there's more of you to hug, and your friends may tease you about your clothes looking tighter. It's difficult indeed to imagine someone asking, "What are you trying to do, give yourself diabetes?" We don't usually make a mental connection between obesity and diabetes.

And yet that one connection is probably the single most important reason that diabetes is so widespread within the African-American community. On the average, black folks are significantly heavier than whites. While 25 percent of Americans as a whole are obese, obesity affects over 30 percent of African-Americans. Among black young adults (age twenty-five to thirty-four), 20 percent of men and 33 percent of women are overweight. As we get older, we get heavier. That's especially true for black women; by middle age, more than 60 percent of our mothers and sisters and aunts meet the clinical definition of overweight.

How fat is "obese"? Doctors measure obesity against so-called ideal weights. These numbers, based largely on information from life insurance companies, reflect the fact that people who weigh too much have a greater-than-average risk of dying before their time. Insurance tables have been around for quite some time, long enough for people to grow critical of them. For one thing, the insurance records used to generate average weights come from white middle-class males. Critics have charged that because the insurance records reflect a narrow segment of the population at large, ideal weight tables aren't valid for anyone but white middle-class males. The tables also don't allow for age—an important distinction, since people typically gain weight when they grow older. Even the United States Centers for Disease Control (CDC) has publicly questioned the validity of ideal-weight tables.

In 1990 these and other criticisms helped prod the federal government into releasing a new table of ideal weights that is much more generous than previous guides.

HOW MUCH SHOULD YOU WEIGH?

HEIGHT (WITHOUT SHOES)	WEIGHT (MEN OR WOMEN) (WITHOUT SHOES)	
	Age 19 to 34	Age 35 and up
5'0"	97–128	108–138
5'1"	101–132	111–143
5'2"	104–137	115–148
5'3"	107–141	119–152
5'4"	111–146	122–157
5'5"	114–150	126–162
5'6"	118–155	130–167
5'7"	121–160	134–172
5'8"	125–164	138–178
5'9"	129–169	142–183
5'10"	132–174	146–188
5'11"	136–179	151–194
6'0"	140–184	155–199
6'1"	144–189	159–205
6'2"	148–195	164–210
6'3"	152–200	168–216

SOURCE: Dietary Guidelines for Americans, 1990.

Even by these more generous definitions, many African-Americans find themselves pushing the upper end of what's considered healthy body weight. That's especially true for black women. And so it shouldn't be surprising that black women also face a high rate of diabetes—even higher than black men.

When it comes to diabetes, experts tell us that all obesity is not alike. Two people who weigh the same number of pounds can wind up with different risks of developing diabetes. That's because what counts is not just how much you weigh, but where the weight is located. If your fat is distributed mostly above your waist, your chances of developing diabetes are higher than if your body fat is positioned below your waist. Obesity specialists sometimes talk of "apple" physiques and "pear" physiques. These terms refer to the two major types of body fat distribution.

There's actually an easy way to calculate whether you classify as an apple or a pear. Using a tape measure, measure your abdomen at its largest point. Then measure your hips at their widest point. Now divide the first number by the second number. For example, if your waist measures 36 inches and your hips measure 40 inches, the waist-to-hips ratio is 36 divided by 40, or .9.

This represents a low diabetes risk, according to a team of endocrinologists at the Louisiana State Medical Center. Working with women through the Charity Hospital System, the researchers discovered that diabetics had high waist-to-hips ratios (average ratio .954) while nondiabetics had low ratios (average .895). In other words, people who have lots of upper-body fat (the apple physique) are more prone to diabetes than are people whose body fat is distributed like a pear. In fact, says obesity expert Dr. F. Xavier Pi-Sunyer of Columbia University, "Obesity in the upper body...carries the risk not only for diabetes but for hypertension, coronary vascular disease [heart disease], and stroke. Lower-body obesity is much less risky."

As it turns out, the abdominal fat of "apples" is much more active metabolically than is the hip and thigh fat of "pears." Abdominal fat is mobile; it readily moves from the fat cells, where it's stored, into the bloodstream. There it stimulates the liver to break down glycogen into glucose, which in turn spills into the bloodstream and begins to raise blood glucose levels. This wouldn't be a problem for a healthy person. All the pancreas would have to do is crank out a little insulin, and the glucose would stream from the bloodstream into the body's tissues. But because hefty people are resistant to insulin, their bodies aren't very responsive to insulin. That means it's harder for them to rid their arteries of excess glucose. Suddenly, Type 2 diabetes is just around the corner.

If you're an overweight adult, see your doctor and ask to be tested for diabetes. According to an expert panel of the National Institutes of Health, all overweight adults are at risk of diabetes. That goes doubly for African-Americans, because our weight is just one of many reasons why we're at risk of diabetes.

POVERTY

We raise de wheat,
Dey gib us de corn;
We bake de bread,
Dey gib us de crust;
We sif de meal,
Dey gib us de huss;
We peel de meat,
Dey gib us de skin;
And dat's de way
Dey take us in;
We skim de pot,
Dey gib us de liquor,
And say dat's good enough for the nigger.

When abolitionist Frederick Douglass wrote the folk song, "We Raise de Wheat," in 1853, Franklin Pierce was President, California was entering the Union, and the *New York Times* had just hit the streets for a penny a copy. The times were wholly different than they are today. And yet for black Americans, the denial of opportunity that Douglass wrote about 140 years ago is still very much a part of daily life. Nearly one third of all African-Americans live below the poverty line, and millions more have just enough money to disqualify them from social programs but not nearly enough to make a dent in the inequity that surrounds them.

What does poverty mean for African-Americans? For one thing, it means limited access to quality health care. Back when public facilities were still segregated, there were over four hundred black hospitals at one time or another from coast to coast. Today that number has dwindled to around twenty-five. In their place has sprung a legion of private hospitals. But these have largely relocated to the suburbs in search of affluent customers, thereby abandoning the inner city where our community needs them the most. And many of the private doctors who still practice near low-income African-Americans refuse to treat them. "Because Medicaid reimbursement levels are so low," writes Harlem Hospital pediatrician Dr. Margaret Heagerty in the *Journal of Health Care for the Poor and Underserved*, "and probably because of social class biases and racism, most physicians in the private sector elect not to provide care for Medicaid patients, never mind those without insurance." (According to federal statistics, one in four black Americans, and 35 percent of poor blacks, have neither public nor private health insurance.) That means that large numbers of inner-city African-Americans must rely on a public health care system that, particularly since the massive federal cutbacks of the 1980s, is notorious for long waiting lines, crowded clinics, inconvenient locations, overworked staffs, and sometimes callous attitudes.

Even in rural areas, African-Americans find it difficult to get the health care we need. We like to think of country living as carefree, but anyone who has ever lived in a remote area appreciates the risks of rural life, particularly in the rural South. Distance determines the availability of health care in rural America. In Tennessee, for example, thirty-five of the state's seventy-five counties lack even a single obstetrician, and if you are too poor to own a car, you are forced to fend for yourself. Throughout the South many thousands of poor black families live in substandard housing, send their children to inadequate schools, and earn so little money that meaningful health care, even if it were nearby, would be unaffordable. And so people get sick and die young. "Rural children born in Mississippi are at greater risk of dying during the first year of life than are their urban counterparts in any other state," says Dr. L. C. Dorsey of Delta Health Center in Mound Bayou, Mississippi. "Rural African-American children in Mississippi are twice as likely to die during the first year of life than are their white counterparts." No matter where you live, if you're poor and black, it's much harder to stay healthy.

One of the best examples is diabetes. For starters, poor people have more diabetes. Body weight is one reason why. On the average, poor people are more obese than more affluent people are and, as we've seen, folks who are fat are at risk of diabetes. Once someone has the disease, misinformation about diabetes and a lack of affordable care contribute to a higher rate of medical complications, like end-stage renal disease. When those complications set in, poor patients find that the medical tools for treating diabetes—pancreas transplants, laser surgery for eyes, kidney dialysis, and even certain medicines—are prohibitively expensive. As Dr. David Stern of the University of Texas Health Science Center told the *New York Times*, "You're going to face more problems if you run out of medicine because you don't have the money." And Uncle Sam doesn't always pick up the tab. "On my limited income, I have to have some help," thirty-year-old Mary Lynn Williams, diabetic since the age of nine, told the *Atlanta Constitution*. "Medicaid is not enough for all the medicine I need."

Of course, it's one thing to be frustrated in treating a disease that you know you have. Plenty of black folks don't even know they have diabetes. In Georgia, where the Diabetes Association of Atlanta reaches out to low-income people with free insulin, needles, and other aid, counseling and education are among the two most important services a poor person can receive. "There are many people who are undiagnosed diabetics that are in need of assistance," one physician explained to the *Atlanta Constitution*. "The public health sector has barely scratched the surface in reaching them." The longer someone has diabetes without it being diagnosed, the easier it is for the disease to progress to an advanced stage and the more difficult it is to treat. Ultimately, diabetics who don't know they have diabetes are setting themselves up for disaster.

It's important to understand that all of us, whether we're rich or poor, urban or suburban or rural, can do a great many things to protect ourselves from diabetes and a number of other diseases. Poverty doesn't doom a person to diabetes any more than wealth makes them immune to it. But the fact that so many African-Americans are indeed poor is one of the principal reasons that we wrestle with so many cases of diabetes, and one of the reasons that overcoming diabetes takes harder work.

LACK OF EXERCISE

It's a raw winter evening, your job has been eight hours of wall-to-wall frustration, and the only thing that will salvage the day is your favorite comfort food: a steaming plate of black-eyed peas and rice. Do you: 1) pick up the phone and order a plate from Mama's Soul Food Emporium; 2) reach into the freezer and try to locate leftovers from your last comfort-food splurge; or 3) dust off your cookbook and make dinner from scratch?

No matter which option you would choose, you'd still save an amazing amount of work over the traditional way. Planting, weeding, harvesting, shelling, threshing, grinding—it all took such prodigious patience and muscles that most of us today hardly consider farming our food a realistic option.

Yet our ancestors had no choice. These resilient women and men received so much exercise satisfying the sweaty demands of daily life that they didn't have to worry about staying in shape. They didn't have to worry about diabetes, either. Their active lifestyles helped protect them. (Some scientists say the strenuous exercise of farming and other outdoor activities helps explain why rural men have little diabetes even today.)

But once blacks left southern farms for the urban North, they began to leave behind a vigorous, demanding lifestyle and enter an age of convenience. Suddenly there were automobiles instead of horses and buggies, and neighborhood markets instead of farms. Many felt that labor-saving devices would raise America to the pinnacle of western advancement. As early as 1853, one American periodical, the *U.S. Review*, had announced that machinery would eventually do all of our work, freeing people to love, study, and be happy. It hasn't quite worked out that way, of course. At least not yet. But nobody can argue that the western lifestyle, with its emphasis on technology and gadgets, has contributed to a sharp decline in the amount of exercise that we get. This in turn has hastened the proliferation of diabetes. (We'll explore the link between exercise and diabetes in Chapter 7.)

The exercise/diabetes connection is directly relevant to African-Americans. Whereas most white Americans don't get enough exercise, blacks may get even less. That's the word from the University of Pittsburgh, where scientists took a close look at why black women weigh more than white women. It wasn't that black women in the study ate more; both groups consumed the same number of calories. The difference was black women exercised less. They walked less, they climbed fewer stairs, they played fewer sports. If these findings are valid for blacks across the board, then physical activity—or lack of it—could be another reason why so many African-Americans become diabetic.

IS DIABETES INEVITABLE?

It's natural to ponder whether African-Americans are somehow destined to get diabetes. As you consider the evidence, you might even find yourself a little confused. For example, it's a well-known fact that diabetes runs in the family. If your parents have it, for example, you're likely to have it. On the other hand, as we can see by the low rates of diabetes in traditional Africa, there's nothing about African-Americans' genes that make our race prone to diabetes. If that's the case, you might wonder, then how can it be transmitted from generation to generation?

That may be where other factors step in. For instance, we know that the tendency toward obesity is often passed on from one generation to the next. That doesn't mean that all black children will grow up to be fat. It does mean that children whose parents are hefty have a greater risk than others of growing up heavy themselves. Poverty can run from one generation to the next; many of us know first-hand how difficult it is to break the cycle of poverty. And lifestyles, which are often related to family custom and habits, follow generational lines as well.

So even though nobody has discovered a gene that would link diabetes with African-Americans, our risk of the disease is strong

and related to important factors that tend to cycle from one generation to the next. But don't for an instant assume that our community is powerless against diabetes. Diabetes is a serious disease, but
it's a disease that we can fight. The next five chapters explain how.

SO YOU'VE GOT "SUGAR"

A few years ago a Chicago hospital had a patient who was so unusual that doctors, nurses, even the housekeeping staff dropped by his room to see for themselves the miracle that people were talking about. His name was Thomas Goldston, a black real estate developer who had been found in a coma and rushed to Michael Reese Hospital and Medical Center, his blood sugar a remarkable sixteen times higher than normal. Though Goldston was a diabetic, he was casual about his lifestyle—he admits he was a heavy drinker—and he resisted seeking medical care. "I just didn't want to believe I was sick," he told *Ebony*. "And I didn't want to be bothered with seeing doctors all the time."

Goldston saw plenty of doctors once he was hospitalized. He had lost so much fluid that his dehydrated brain barely kept him alive. Doctors didn't expect him to survive, but after being in a coma for nearly a month, Goldston gradually regained his faculties. Today Thomas Goldston is a changed man. He takes insulin like clockwork, he exercises regularly, he eats right, and he monitors his urine and blood at home for glucose. "I'm trying to do the right thing, not only because my doctor fusses with me when I don't but also because I'm fighting for my life."

Goldston's story is unusual because of what happened: few

diabetics recover from such a dire emergency. But *why* it happened, unfortunately, is all too common. Goldston was one of millions of African-American diabetics who take their disease too casually. They ignore the fact that their relatives have diabetes. Then they shrug off warning signs that diabetes is upon them. Before they know it, the disease has advanced, they're in excruciating pain, and saving their kidneys or toes or legs—or their very lives—has become a desperate race against the clock.

Goldston was lucky. Most people in his position are not. That's why it's extremely important to forge a partnership with your doctor, get the very best medical care that you can, and follow your doctor's advice.

Many black folks are reluctant to do this. Instead of actively seeking out medical care, we resist it. Dr. Ghassan Hamadeh, who spent time treating black diabetics on South Carolina's Sea Islands, noticed one attitude that prevails in many black communities across the country. "Some blacks in the Sea Islands have a belief that going to the hospital means the end of their life," says Hamadeh. "Seeing the physician means that one is close to death."

The roots of these and other health beliefs may be deeply imbedded in our culture. Medical historian Dr. Todd Savitt of the East Carolina University School of Medicine says nineteenth-century medicine was crude—and slaves knew it. "They knew that physicians...were severely limited in the amount of good they could do. Because no one understood the etiology [cause] of most diseases, no one could effectively cure them." Not only were typical remedies ineffective, they were often harsh. They also clashed with African beliefs that illnesses are cured by deities and ancestors, not pills and potions.

Slaves' mistrust of the white man's cures, and their unwillingness to surrender their bodies to an unfamiliar system of medicine, made them reluctant to report illnesses until various home remedies—herbs, roots, prayer—had been exhausted. Home care was easy to learn—"anyone could practice blood-letting or dosing with a little experience," says Savitt—and stocking a home medicine chest was considerably less expensive than paying for a doctor's services. In times of illness, slaves also summoned local black healers. Conjurers worked their magic and root doctors brought their concoctions. Only when home cures failed did the typical slave convey word of an illness to the slavemaster, who, concerned about losing his investment, would summon a doctor. But because many plantations were located in remote areas, and horseback was the fastest means of transportation, long hours often passed before the physician's arrival. By then a slave could be on death's door.

So you see, there are historical reasons that many black folks say seeing a doctor means the end of the road—not too long ago it often *was* the end of the road. Our experience during slavery also sheds light on other present-day behaviors, including mistrust of modern medicine and reliance on home remedies and neighborhood healers.

Belief in tradition is soothing and necessary. All of us need to understand where we came from, and we all need to respect the ways of those who have come before us. But as a physician who has repeatedly witnessed the tragic consequences of people delaying to seek care, and of relying on traditional methods that can be ineffective if not harmful, I respectfully call on black Americans to consider a more reliable approach. It starts with finding out if you have diabetes.

What are the symptoms of diabetes?

There are twelve classic warning signs of Type 2 diabetes—the kind that most black diabetics have:

1. Skin, gum, or bladder infections that recur or are hard to heal
2. Drowsiness
3. Blurred vision
4. Tingling or numbness in hands or feet
5. Itchy skin
6. Frequent urination
7. Excessive thirst
8. Extreme hunger
9. Dramatic weight loss
10. Irritability
11. Weakness and fatigue
12. Nausea and vomiting

Symptoms six through twelve are also warning signs for Type 1 diabetes.

In Type 1 diabetes the symptoms are usually sudden and severe. In Type 2 the symptoms are gradual and less striking. For example, while a person with Type 1 diabetes may have to urinate urgently twenty-four hours a day, someone with Type 2 diabetes may have to do so only after dark. You can see why Type 2 diabetes is often deceptive. "The disease can really creep up on you," one forty-seven-year-old school principal told a *Time* magazine reporter after suffering an amputation and a stroke from what started as "just a mild case of diabetes." In the early stages, the disease may not have any symptoms at all. And yet that's the time to act. The earlier you treat diabetes, the easier it is to stop it in its tracks. So if you're at risk for diabetes, don't wait until you have symptoms to be examined by a physician.

How can you tell if you're at risk? Years ago doctors found it difficult to predict who would get diabetes. Estimating whether someone would develop the disease "is something that has been tried in the past but was not very successful," Dr. Ronald Kahn of Boston's Joslin Clinic explained to a *New York Times* reporter. But new research suggests that some early signs of diabetes can occur decades before the full-fledged disease. If you're vulnerable to the disease and you and your doctor stay alert for tell-tale signs, you can nip small problems in the bud before they become major ones. You are at risk if you are an African-American and:

1. You are overweight; or
2. There are diabetics in your family; or
3. You have unexplained abnormal nerve sensations (numbness, tingling, pain); or
4. You are over forty years of age.

If you fit one or more of these four categories, go to your doctor once a year and asked to be screened for diabetes. If you are a woman, I also think it's a good idea to be screened if:

1. You have ever given birth to a baby weighing nine pounds or more; or

2. You have had diabetes only during pregnancy; or
3. You have ever had an unexplained spontaneous abortion.

What does screening entail? It involves measuring a blood sample for glucose, and testing a urine sample for glucose and chemicals known as ketones. High glucose levels or the presence of ketones may suggest a potential problem. If this is the case, your doctor should arrange to have you tested for diabetes.

How is diabetes diagnosed?

The standard test for diabetes is called a *glucose tolerance test.* Here's how it works.

Preparation for the test starts a few days beforehand. For at least three days, you will be asked to eat whatever you please as long as it contains at least two hundred grams of carbohydrates per day. (You can use the food exchange lists in Chapter 6 to plan your meals.) Aside from your diet, you do not have to alter your normal activities during these three days. You must fast overnight for ten to twelve hours before the test, although you may drink water.

On the day of the test, you will be asked to drink a beverage of citrus-flavored glucose in water. Someone will draw your blood immediately, then again after thirty minutes, one hour, two hours, and three hours. That's all there is to it. Besides the five needle pricks, some say the most difficult part of the entire ordeal is swallowing the drink. With one hundred grams of glucose, the equivalent of over six tablespoons of table sugar, it is intensely sweet.

The purpose of the blood test is to see how your body handles a sudden influx of sugar. Normally the pancreas responds by using insulin to clear the sugar out of the bloodstream. Nondiabetics typically start the glucose tolerance test with a blood glucose level under 115. Over the next two hours, the glucose level reaches an upper limit of 200. Then as insulin kicks in, the glucose level falls to under 140. Diabetics have difficulty clearing glucose from the blood. If you have diabetes, your blood glucose level is usually over 140 at the start of the test. It rises to over 200 during the test and remains there as long as two hours later. (These numbers are different for children and pregnant women.)

Lots of factors can influence the results of the glucose tolerance test, and your doctor should discuss them with you before the test. Infections (especially if accompanied by a fever), prolonged physical inactivity, and a number of diseases can alter the test results. So can certain antihypertension medicines, hormones (including birth control pills), and other drugs. Your doctor may ask you to stop taking these preparations for the duration of the test. If your doctor thinks that any of these factors may have interfered with the results of the test, you may be asked to repeat it. This should happen at least a week later, to give you—and your body—a chance to recuperate.

In most patients the test results are black and white; either you clearly have diabetes or you don't. In some people the diagnosis will be less clear. For instance, the test may show an elevation in blood glucose that's somewhat higher than normal but not high enough to definitively signal diabetes. Or your doctor's guidelines for how to interpret the test may change. National and international diabetes experts meet periodically to discuss the glucose tolerance test and how it should be interpreted. Sometimes the consensus changes because of new medical evidence. Thus test results that indicated diabetes five or ten years ago might not indicate diabetes today.

I mention these points only to emphasize that because medicine is an evolving science, an accurate diagnosis depends on the experience and wisdom of the practitioner. Some doctors perform the glucose tolerance test improperly, I'm afraid, and others may not know the latest guidelines for interpreting the results. One of the reasons I'm spelling out what the test entails is so you can judge whether your doctor is providing you with quality care.

If a doctor says you have diabetes without having given you a glucose tolerance test, should you believe him or her? Under certain circumstances, yes. Most diabetics have a fasting blood sugar level of over 140. If on two occasions your doctor finds this high level of glucose in your blood, a glucose tolerance test won't be needed to tell that you have diabetes.

What if the test says I have diabetes?

The most common reaction to a diagnosis of diabetes is profound shock. If you have a diabetic relative, you may find yourself unable to think of anything but their amputated toe or leg. If you're a parent you may feel guilty, as if you were somehow responsible for your child's diabetes, and you may wonder how you'll be able to care for a child with such a serious disease. Elders already struggling with other chronic diseases may feel overwhelmed with the added burden of coping with one more. Athletes may wonder if they'll have to give up sports. People who are unattached may worry about their chances of finding a partner, and young women may wonder if the disease will prevent them from having a child.

This is a diagnosis that turns people's worlds upside down. One journalist who was diagnosed as diabetic as a college student remembers the sensation clearly. "While my housemates were consuming ice cream or pizza with abandon at 3 A.M., I anxiously measured food by the gram on a tiny scale, trying to adhere to the American Diabetes Association's strict dietary regimen," he wrote in *Health* magazine. "Ahead of me, I thought, was a life of being 'different': no travel, no girlfriends. I felt like my world was imploding."

Bewilderment, disbelief, anxiety—these are all common reactions to the diagnosis of diabetes. You may feel powerless against a disease that has no cure, and you may despair at the prospect of medical complications. Diabetes demands that people attend to their body's needs very closely, and if you're not used to watching your health or you're not very disciplined, the thought of testing your blood like clockwork or injecting yourself with insulin every day can be extremely difficult to accept. Sometimes the diagnosis brings out people's worst fears. One diabetic confided in Boston psychiatrist Dr. David Holmes this frightening scenario: "After I become blind, my gangrenous limbs will be amputated and I shall be totally dependent on others. Ultimately, people will withdraw. In the end, I shall be helpless and friendless, in strange surroundings."

Things usually don't work out that way, of course. Diabetics and the people who love them learn to adjust to the disease, and a person's worst fears never materialize. But these and other concerns that arise from the initial shock of diagnosis should be discussed, not suppressed. Talking with family and friends, or sitting down with a trusted older relative or minister, may help you sort through these difficult feelings. If you feel utterly unable to cope, or if you find that being diagnosed as a diabetic has stirred up troubling feelings that you don't know to handle, psychotherapy or psychiatric counseling can be very helpful.

Diabetes will bring new changes to your life. Accepting that fact can be difficult, but it can be done. Consider it the first major hurdle of this new phase of your life. Leaping it successfully will pave the way for other successes in monitoring your condition and making sure your body has what it needs to be healthy.

Once you are diagnosed, you should receive a thorough medical exam. The idea is to find out how advanced the diabetes is and whether it is impairing any part of your body. The exam can take place in a doctor's office, in a clinic, or in a hospital.

What will the doctor do?

Diabetes is a complex condition, so if your doctor is good, she or he will take a fair amount of time to make sure every base is covered. For starters the doctor should inquire about your history. At a bare minimum, these are the sorts of questions you should be asked, according to Boston's Joslin Clinic:

- When did you first begin to notice any symptoms?
- Do any members of your family have diabetes?
- What kinds of health problems have members of your family experienced?
- What illnesses and hospitalizations have you had, and when did they occur?
- Are you taking any medications? What are they? What dosage?

If you are seeing a doctor by appointment, many offices ask patients to fill out a questionnaire in advance. This gives the patient a chance to consult with family members to ensure that the information being supplied is accurate.

Next comes a complete physical exam. The doctor should examine your eyes and test your nerves. Blood pressure is such an important indicator of the risk of diabetic complications that it should be measured three ways: when you are lying down, sitting up, and standing. This is because your blood pressure changes depending on body position. Your feet should be very carefully examined for signs of infection. The doctor should check your circulation by feeling for your pulse in your feet and legs. Women should receive pelvic examinations; everyone should get a rectal exam. Since diabetes affects body weight, your weight should be carefully measured and recorded, along with your height. This is especially important if the patient is a child or an adolescent; accurate records will give the doctor a baseline for future comparison with nondiabetic youngsters.

Your doctor should order several lab tests. You will be asked to give samples of urine and blood so they can be tested for glucose. The doctor should also take a blood count. The tests for glucose are extremely important and the doctor should ideally be located close enough to a lab to receive the results of these tests during the first appointment.

What should the doctor tell me?

Patient education is a big part of managing diabetes successfully. Diabetics need to know not only how sick they are, but what they need to do—in very specific language—to preserve their health. Your doctor should explain what the various tests reveal and what your new responsibilities as a diabetic are.

If you have Type 1 diabetes, your doctor will prescribe insulin to compensate for your body's inability to produce the hormone. If you have Type 2 diabetes, you will be asked to lose weight, usually by eating well and exercising. If good eating and regular exercise don't produce the intended weight loss, the doctor may prescribe insulin, or tablets or pills that stimulate your body to make insulin, or both. (More on these later.) Whichever course will be pursued, your doctor should explain the treatment and what it will mean for you to comply with it.

That first session may last an hour or so. During that time your doctor may introduce you to a nurse or a dietitian. These health professionals should instruct you on the following:

- What diabetes is and how it affects the body
- How to monitor your blood and urine at home
- How to manage your diet
- How to use insulin (if the doctor prescribes it)
- How to eat, keep up with your insulin, and test your urine on days that you are sick
- How to take care of your teeth, feet, and skin

HOW TO CHOOSE A DIABETES DOCTOR

If your car needed a specialized part—a certain clamp, for instance—and you asked for it at your corner gas station, you probably wouldn't have much luck. It would be far better to visit a mechanic who specializes in servicing your specific make and model of car.

But millions of diabetics receive treatment from generalists—family doctors, internists, general practitioners—who aren't always familiar with the latest research. That's the word from *McCall's* magazine, which reports that these doctors sometimes make mistakes, anything from failing to test for glycosylated hemoglobin, a bloodstream chemical that's elevated in diabetics to neglecting to advise a patient to monitor their blood and urine for glucose.

Make sure this doesn't happen to you. If you have a choice about which doctor you will see (patients at public clinics often have little say in who treats them), ask a nurse or doctor for a recommendation. Look for a physician who has a good reputation and who has treated a number of diabetics. A good doctor:

- Explains the fundamentals of diabetes clearly and simply, and either refers you to sources of more information or gives you printed material to take home. Some doctors simply hand patients a piece of paper explaining their new diet. That's not enough.

- Is specific. Instead of saying "Your blood pressure is a little high," a good doctor explains, "Your blood pressure is 160/100. Let's try to get it down to 140/80."

- Reviews your home blood-sugar records and backs them up with glycosylated hemoglobin tests.

- Keeps a watchful eye for complications by regularly checking your blood pressure and cholesterol and examining your feet.

- Refers you to an ophthalmologist for eye testing.

You should also receive instructions on when and where you should make follow-up visits.

If this session takes place on the same day as your diagnosis, you may find yourself so stunned by the news that it's difficult to let much of what the doctor says sink in. Good physicians understand this and take care to present information clearly and simply, repeating it if necessary. By the same token, if you are confused about what you are hearing, speak up. If there are things that you don't understand, ask questions. Don't be reluctant to assert your needs. Health professionals are paid to present information in a way that you can understand it. If you leave the office without a clear understanding of your condition and what you should do about it, they're not doing their job.

What's my prognosis?

Once you have been diagnosed as diabetic, it's only natural to wonder about the long-term consequences. On this point the news for black Americans is not entirely grim. You'll recall that diabetes is more prevalent in the black community than among whites. Black people also suffer more complications of diabetes. Compared to whites, we have more visual impairment, more end-stage renal disease, and more amputations. Yet once we have diabetes, we seem to die from it at slightly lower rates. That's according to a 1990 National Institutes of Health study that found diabetes mentioned on 3 percent of death certificates for whites but only 2 percent of death certificates for blacks. The difference may seem small, but considering what we're up against, I think it's a minor miracle.

Longevity is among a diabetic's most urgent concerns. Many diabetics hold fluctuating expectations of the future, says psychiatrist Dr. David Holmes, "from an unexamined sense that they will live happily ever after, to the equally unrealistic notion that they will drop dead in a moment." Dr. Holmes tells of an eighteen-year-old diabetic who, after entering college and discovering that she was merely one of a number of bright people, became fixated on the finite nature of her existence. Having already established her own probable life expectancy, she revised her estimate from age forty-nine to age thirty-nine. Then she happened to form a close

AVOID THESE DIABETES "TREATMENTS"

Each year, Americans fork over $2.24 billion for what the government calls "questionable treatments" for diabetes and other serious chronic ailments. Given African-Americans' distrust of western medicine and the traditional African belief that illness is caused and cured by spirits, we may be more tempted to invest our hard-earned dollars in treatments that have never been proven effective.

Take bee pollen, for example. Some people believe that diabetics benefit by eating flower pollen collected by bees and stored in the hive for food. "It's supposedly the thing the queen bee eats that makes her grow and gives her special strength," said Frank Robles, former president of the Utah chapter of the American Diabetes Association in an interview with the *Wall Street Journal.* The only problem is that people aren't bees. There's no evidence that bee pollen does much to benefit humans. In fact, if you have allergies to flowering plants, such a concentrated dose of pollen can kick off a severe allergic reaction.

Some diabetics believe that juniper berries can help control the disease. What they often don't realize is that these small berries are 30 percent sugar—not the best thing for someone on a low-sugar diet.

Some people who advocate iridology—the practice of examining the iris of the eye for light and dark spots in an attempt to diagnose illness—might prescribe any number of herbal treatments for diabetes. Then after several visits, the iridologist may discover that the treatment "worked" and the spots have disappeared. Iridology is a lot like astrology, says Robles. It can be used any way the practitioner wants.

If you've got a few thousand dollars to burn and you don't mind traveling halfway across the globe, you can even have your diabetic pancreas "removed" in the Philippines. That's where con artists called faith healers use sleight of hand to create the illusion that they are removing a damaged organ—all without actually opening the skin. "It's all chicken parts and coagulated blood," says Frank Robles.

These remedies do little but prey on your hope—and wallet. Sometimes they can even hurt your health. My advice: steer clear of them.

friendship with another woman and in so doing because less anxious about her disease. Her pessimism diminished somewhat and she revised her estimate again from age thirty-nine to age fifty.

Little is known about the longevity of African-American diabetics. But we can find some clues from examining statistics on white diabetics. For whites (mostly Type 1 diabetics) diagnosed with diabetes before age thirty, the disease has a rather startling impact on overall life expectancy, according to Joslin Center records. The average Type 1 diabetic dies at age fifty for women and age forty-eight for men. (This compares to the average life expectancy in the general population of seventy-eight years for women and seventy-two years for men.)

For people (mostly Type 2 diabetics) diagnosed after age thirty, the picture is a little brighter. The average life expectancy climbs to sixty-five for women and sixty-six for men.

Black Americans as a whole can expect to live an average of five to seven fewer years than whites. The reasons are varied: poorer access to health care, inferior quality of care, a shortage of health professionals willing to practice in underserved black communities, too little emphasis on prevention. But even though it's more difficult for African-Americans to be healthy, black people still own the keys to good health. That's because when it comes to becoming healthy and staying healthy, one of the most important factors is your attitude—your willingness to do what's best for your health. And no one can take that away from you.

Let me give you an example. While thumbing through the archives of the *Journal of the National Medical Association*, I found a disturbing case about a black physician who was brought to the hospital in a coma with a badly gangrenous foot. The year was 1937, long after the discovery of insulin and a time when many of today's principles for treating diabetes were already in use. Nevertheless, this sixty-three-year-old woman had failed to take her disease seriously. "She had known about the existence of diabetes for some time but instituted no treatment until about two weeks before entrance into the hospital," wrote the doctor in charge of the case. Her blood sugar was high—340 compared to the normal 115 or less—and she had acetone in her urine. With treatment, the woman recovered. But it was too late to save her leg, which was amputated shortly thereafter. As she was recovering from surgery, she died of pneumonia.

You would expect a black physician, of all people, to respect the devastation that diabetes can cause. But in the end, this unfortunate woman became just another statistic. Like millions of African-Americans, she failed to seize the initiative. She waited until it was too late to take care of herself, and the results were devastating. The same thing nearly happened with Thomas Goldston, the Chicago real estate investor who nearly lost his life in a diabetic coma.

It shouldn't take a brush with death to motivate us to care for ourselves. The fact is, diabetics have plenty of motivation for taking charge of their health and closely following their doctor's instructions: diabetics who do this live longer and suffer fewer complications. They have fewer hospital bills. Their quality of life is better. And in my experience, they are also happier and better able to function in the world.

To reap these many benefits, you need several things. First of all, you need to know you have diabetes. Only about half of all black Americans who have diabetes know they are diabetics. The rest live with a smoldering disease that could be making them sicker each year without their knowing why. So if your doctor has said you have diabetes, you already you have an advantage over your less fortunate brothers and sisters: you know what you're up against.

Second, you have to accept the fact that merely knowing the diagnosis isn't enough. That black physician knew she had diabetes, too, but she didn't do anything about it. Once you realize you have diabetes, you must act on it. It's the best way—the only way—to ensure a long and happy life.

OK! I'm willing to accept my diabetes and take charge of my health. What's the next step?

The next step is to learn new skills and begin new habits. Unlike even a decade or two ago, diabetics today can live near-normal lives. But you have to know what your body needs. Even more important, you have to be willing to provide it. Let's start with a few of the basics of living with diabetes.

LIVING WITH DIABETES

Hardy Franklin knows diabetes like a book. And that's saying a lot, because if there's one thing Hardy Franklin knows, it's books. Franklin, a black man, is the sixty-three-year-old president of the American Library Association. He has lived successfully with diabetes for the past twenty-one years, and he's done it by being smart. He exercises regularly and takes his insulin three times a day, testing his blood sugar before each dose. "Like my mother [who had Type 1 diabetes], I am careful of my diabetes," Franklin told the American Diabetes Association. "I eat at regular hours, and, like her, I know fried foods and desserts are a thing of the past."

As a diabetic, you will learn how to give your body the food, the exercise, and (if your doctor prescribes it) the medication you need to be healthy. The goal behind all three is to control your blood sugar. This makes sense. After all, the reason you have diabetes is that your pancreas has lost touch with the rest of the tissues in your body, and insulin no longer efficiently removes sugar from your blood. By eating well, exercising, and taking medicine, you encourage your body to carry glucose from your bloodstream to the rest of your body just as it would normally.

Thus taking charge of diabetes means gently coaxing your body back into a healthy pattern of glucose management. Managing your blood glucose not only helps you feel better in the short-term, by avoiding the immediate side effects of blood sugar that is too low; it also helps you avoid the long-term complications of blood sugar that's too high—losing your eyesight, suffering an amputation, going into kidney failure, or worse. "There's a general perception that excessive glucose is the primary culprit in complications," Dr. Harry Shamoon of New York City's Albert Einstein College of Medicine told *Health* magazine.

Whether you have Type 1 or Type 2 diabetes, the idea is to mimic the blood sugar levels you would have if your pancreas and other tissues functioned normally. That's where exercise, diet, and medicine come in. Food raises your blood glucose level. Exercise lowers it. Insulin and insulin-stimulating medicines lower it as well. You can use these three tools to make sure your blood sugar is neither too high nor too low. Your job as captain of the ship is to steer a middle ground where your body is happiest.

Of course, every captain needs a compass to help them stay on course. For diabetics that compass is a device that monitors your blood for glucose.

WHAT IS BLOOD MONITORING ALL ABOUT?

Monitoring your blood is easy. All it takes is a blood glucose monitoring kit, which you can buy over the counter at pharmacies and some supermarkets. There are a number of monitoring kits on the market, but the essential elements are 1) a meter for measuring the glucose; 2) test strips to hold a sample of blood; and 3) a pricking device to draw the blood sample.

To run the test, first you prick a clean finger and place a drop of blood on the pad of a test strip. Then you start the meter. A timer in the meter lets you know when enough time has elapsed for chemicals in the test strip to react with the blood. The meter signals you to blot the excess blood from the test strip. Then the meter signals you to insert the test strip in the meter. A short time later, the meter displays your blood glucose level.

WHAT IS LOW BLOOD SUGAR? ▰▰▰▰▰▰▰▰▰▰

When you don't eat for a while, your body starts to run out of glucose from your last meal. If you have a normal metabolism, hormones come to the rescue. Glucagon sent from your pancreas arrives at your liver, causing the liver to bring glucose out of storage and into the bloodstream. Insulin meets the glucose and carries it into your tissues. Other hormones do their part as well, actually manufacturing glucose from the body's storehouse of proteins and other substances. Thanks to hormones, your body has the continuous supply of blood sugar that it needs.

But if you have diabetes, this hormonal balancing act never gets off the ground. If you're a diabetic and 1) you take too much insulin or diabetes medicine, 2) you go without food after taking insulin injections or diabetes medicine, or 3) you go without food after exercising excessively, your blood sugar can start to fall. Without food or a well-oiled hormonal backup system, there's no glucose to replace the sugar you lose.

The signs of low blood sugar or *hypoglycemia*, listed below, shouldn't be ignored. They mean there's trouble ahead unless prompt action is taken. If blood sugar drops too low, a diabetic can lose consciousness, lapse into a coma, and die.

Irritability	Headache
Shakiness	Inability to concentrate
Nervousness	Slurred speech
Rapid heartbeat	Blurred vision
Hunger	Confusion
Perspiration	Irrational behavior
Paleness	Amnesia
Unusual skin sensations	Severe drowsiness
	Seizures

If you experience any these signs, move quickly. Drink or eat something containing sugar—orange juice, cola, ginger ale, candy, even sugar cubes. The idea is to get sugar into your bloodstream as fast as possible.

If your body is denied sugar without relief, you may get to the point where you lose control over your ability to eat or drink. Your

Continued on page 60

friends and family can help in such a situation. Instruct them ahead of time to use a small spoon or a straw to carefully place a tiny amount of a thick sweet liquid, such as corn syrup, between your cheek and gum. Unlike a thin liquid, which could drip down into your lungs and cause pneumonia, a thick liquid will slide down your throat just as saliva does. It goes without saying that medical care by the fastest means possible is an absolute must.

Some of the newer glucose monitors are even easier. To operate the pocket-sized monitors made by Medisense, Inc., of Waltham, Massachusetts, all you do is insert a test strip in the device and apply a drop of blood. The monitor starts automatically; there are no buttons to push. Twenty seconds later, the device displays your blood glucose level. You don't have to blot the blood or clean the device, because blood stays on the disposable test strip instead of entering the monitor.

MONITORING BLOOD SUGAR THE EASY WAY

Monitoring your blood sugar is becoming more and more convenient. Many monitors are battery-operated. They're small and portable enough to slip into a pocket or purse and go wherever you go. Some models have a memory feature that stores previous blood glucose readings, according to *FDA Consumer*. Some even have built-in modems that transmit readings electronically to your doctor's office.

In the last couple of years, innovative designers have built in features that make these devices even more user-friendly, according to the *Wall Street Journal*. The MediSense Company of Cambridge, Massachusetts, has come out with two meters—one the size of a pen, the other the size of a credit card—that are designed on the premise that diabetics will use monitors more faithfully if they can use them discreetly. And Boehringer Mannheim of Indianapolis, Indiana, has introduced a blood glucose monitor that speaks, leading the user through the test and announcing the blood sugar level. It's designed to help diabetics whose vision is impaired.

Home glucose monitoring has come a long way since it began in the late 1960s. In the old days, diabetics used to measure their urine for the glucose that their kidneys were filtering from the bloodstream. But there were lots of problems with urine monitoring. Urine tests were imprecise, because they measure the sugar that has spilled over from the bloodstream, not the sugar level in the blood itself. And urine testing worked best at measuring only high levels of blood sugar, which meant that you could have a low level and fail to detect it.

When blood glucose monitors came on the scene in the late 1960s, they offered direct measurements of both high and low blood sugar—a clear improvement over the urine test. These monitors typically asked users to dot a chemically treated test strip with

HOW TO CHOOSE A BLOOD SUGAR MONITOR

There are lots of blood sugar monitors on the market these days. But they don't all deliver the same value for your money. When the Food and Drug Administration took a close look at nine meters, they found some difficult to use, others with instructions that were difficult to understand. As a result, when the FDA asked experienced users to try the monitors, two thirds made significant errors.

Here's some advice for shopping for a blood glucose monitor:

- Make sure the labels on the controls and buttons are easy to read.

- If a meter signals the user with a beep, make sure the beep is audible. The FDA found that half of the meters it tested produced beeps that couldn't be heard over a normal conversation five feet away.

- If you can, try changing the batteries. Some meters require a degree of dexterity that makes this routine task quite difficult.

- Make sure you can read the instruction manual. Some are printed in type that's too small.

- Be sure you can understand the instructions. Meter manufacturers don't always explain what to do very clearly. Look for manuals that contain graphics. These are helpful, especially for users with poor reading skills.

HOW TO AVOID ERRORS IN MONITORING

If you're not careful when you monitor your blood for glucose, you can easily get an inaccurate reading. Here are some steps the FDA recommends for getting accurate results.

If you suspect a reading is incorrect:

- Check to see that the meter is calibrated. Meters typically must be adjusted to accommodate each new batch of test strips.
- Try a test with blood from a nondiabetic to see if the meter shows glucose in the normal range. That may give you a clue about whether a certain reading for your blood is correct.
- Call a health professional who specializes in diabetes, or dial the manufacturer of the meter for help. Manufacturers often provide toll-free phone numbers for consumer assistance.

To reduce your errors while monitoring, try these tips:

- Seek out professional guidance. Ask a nurse or your doctor to show you how to use the monitor. Later, ask them to watch you test a blood sample to make sure you are still doing it properly.
- Use fresh test strips.
- Clean your meter frequently.
- Follow the manufacturer's instructions carefully.

blood, then to compare the color of the strip against a range of printed colors, each representing a different glucose level. With the introduction of portable meters to read the test strip, glucose monitoring had come into a new age.

Your doctor may advise you to strive for "tight control" of your glucose levels. That means allowing very little fluctuation in blood glucose from hour to hour, day to day. Scientists think that tight control may be the best way to head off the complications of diabetes, although they won't know for sure until sometime in 1993 with the completion of the Diabetes Control and Complications Trial, a project that's been called the largest diabetes study ever undertaken. If tight control is your goal, it means monitoring your blood glucose like clockwork three or more times a day and making sure your blood sugar lies within a normal range. If your blood sugar is too high, you'll have to lower it by exercising or taking insulin or diabetes pills. If it's too low, you'll need to raise it by reducing your dose of insulin or diabetes pills.

WHAT ELSE SHOULD I REMEMBER?

Many of the habits diabetics should adopt are similar to healthy habits that are good for everyone. The differences emerge from the fact that diabetics are particularly vulnerable to certain dangers. Here's a list of do's and don't's.

DO VISIT YOUR DOCTOR REGULARLY   As a person with diabetes, there's a lot that you can do to help safeguard your health. In fact, when it comes right down to it, you are the first line of defense. Your persistence and patience help determine the course of the disease. Invariably, patients who take an active role in this regard come out on top.

But you can't manage the disease on your own. You need the guidance of a health professional, and a single visit to a doctor isn't enough. Diabetes is a long-term condition, so you need to establish a long-term relationship with a doctor. If you don't like the doctor you have, don't let that be an excuse for not having regular checkups. Find someone you like, and visit as often as the doctor recommends. After your first visit, a doctor may ask you to return in anywhere from one week to six months, depending on the treatment being prescribed for you.

Follow-up visits provide a good chance for you to ask questions, to find out whether you are managing your health properly, and to ask about any new products designed to help diabetics. During these visits, the doctor or another health professional may ask you for the results of your home glucose monitoring, and may review the procedure with you to make sure you are monitoring correctly. The doctor should also check for signs of complications by taking your blood pressure, examining your feet, and so forth.

You may have a blood test to check for glucose or glycosylated hemoglobin, or a urine test to check for glucose and ketones. These are important tests because they are key indicators of whether diabetes is being managed appropriately. Unfortunately, they are tests that black men often fail to receive. In a national survey by the National Institutes of Health, only 60 percent of black male diabetics were tested for blood glucose during office visits (compared to 67 to 71 percent of black women, white women, and white men). The survey also asked how many diabetics had received neither blood nor urine tests. Once again, black men had been tested the least; 32 percent of the black men hadn't gotten either test, compared to 26 percent of white men and 24 percent of black and white women. "There may be some deficit in medical care for black diabetics," NIH concluded with some understatement.

DO GET REGULAR DENTAL EXAMS   Tell your dentist you have diabetes. It will help her or him know to watch for gingivitis and periodontal disease, which are common in diabetics. During your first visit, the dentist should take down detailed information about how well you control diabetes and whether you have experienced any medical complications.

DO GET REGULAR EYE CHECKUPS   If you're a black American over age forty, have your eyes tested every two years. And if you have diabetes, get checked every year. That's according to the National Eye Institute, which in 1992 issued sweeping recommendations designed to stem the rising number of cases of serious eye disease. "Millions of people could be saved from vision loss, even blindness, by following these recommendations," said James Mason, head of the United States Public Health Service.

When you visit the eye doctor, be sure to have a *pupil dilation test*. During this test, the doctor places a few drops of medicine in your eyes. The medicine dilates (opens) your pupils so the doctor can check the retina for signs of diabetic retinopathy or glaucoma. After the exam, the doctor either gives you eye drops to constrict your pupils again, or you can wear sunglasses to protect your eyes from light until the pupils return to their normal size on their own.

The test, which takes about an hour, should be performed by an ophthalmologist (a physician who specializes in eye disorders); most optometrists (eye professionals trained to fit prescription glasses) lack the training to recognize diabetic eye disease.

The pupil dilation test is different from the *eye pressure test* that's routinely used during screenings to detect glaucoma. In the pressure test, an instrument is placed on the cornea to detect a buildup of pressure—a warning sign of glaucoma. The hitch is that the pressure test isn't enough; one survey by the National Eye Institute found that three fourths of high-risk glaucoma patients had recently received pressure tests—tests that obviously were of little use in warning of glaucoma. "What we would like to get across," said Dr. Claude Cowan, ophthalmology chief at Howard University Hospital, "is that screening exams that have been used for many, many years to detect glaucoma are inadequate in many patients."

If you wear hard contact lenses, be careful not to wear them for longer than the recommended interval. Overwearing the lenses can scratch your cornea (the transparent surface of your eye). These scratches do not heal as quickly in diabetics, and there is a risk of long-term problems. Soft contact lenses lower the risk of corneal scratches, but they must be cleaned and handled extremely carefully to avoid contaminating the eye and causing an infection.

DO KEEP AN EYE ON YOUR BLOOD PRESSURE   As challenging as diabetes can be, diabetes plus hypertension can make it worse. High blood pressure hastens the development of kidney failure, hardening and thickening of the arteries, eye problems, and other complications. In fact, when Dr. Ronald Klein at the University of Wisconsin Medical School studied nearly one thousand Type 1 diabetics, he found that their degree of hypertension was a "significant predictor" of whether they would eventually develop diabetic retinopathy, the eye disorder. Whether you have Type 1 or Type 2 diabetes, make sure your doctor checks your blood pressure when you visit for a checkup. And if your doctor suggests ways that you should lower your blood pressure, heed this advice. Untreated hypertension is a killer.

BLOOD PRESSURE GUIDELINES FOR DIABETICS ▬▬▬▬▬▬▬▬▬▬

Hypertension is widespread in the African-American community, and it's a major reason why black Americans die at high rates from stroke and heart disease as well as diabetes. But hypertensive diabetics of all colors may suffer not only because of the effects of the condition, but also because the cutoff level used to judge the danger point for high blood pressure isn't safe enough, at least for youngsters with Type 1 diabetes.

When Dr. Kwame Osei, an assistant professor of internal medicine at Ohio State University, compared Type 1 diabetics to healthy peers of the same age and sex, the diabetics had higher average blood pressure—128/84 to 110/71. But even though these elevated readings were "outrageously high," Osei told *USA Today*, they still didn't cross the government's danger level of 140/90, because the federal limit doesn't consider the special hazard to diabetics of even moderately elevated blood pressure. "So my question is, do we need to wait that long, that is, until the pressure hits the cutoff point, before we do something about it?"

If you have Type 1 diabetes, make sure you know your blood pressure numbers, not just whether your pressure is "high" or "about average." Tell your doctor that you'd like to keep your blood pressure as close to normal as possible, and ask what you can do to achieve that beneficial goal.

DO PAMPER YOUR FEET   Feet get no respect. They support us for our entire lives, but if it weren't for an occasional blister or ingrown toenail, most of us wouldn't pay them much attention at all. "The public's not tuned in to general foot care nor to having a routine foot exam," Dr. Norman Klombers, a podiatrist, told *Prevention* magazine. And when you get a physical, most physicians examine every part of you except your feet. "It's as if your body stops just above the ankles," says Dr. Klombers.

Diabetics can't afford to take their feet so casually. The dangers of infection are too great. Here are some steps toward proper foot care:

- Inspect your feet every day. Ask someone else to do it if your eyesight is poor. Diabetics often develop a combination of poor circulation, which slows healing of cuts and infections, and nerve damage, which causes a loss of sensation. Only by checking your feet every day can you catch problems early on. Build a time for foot care into your daily routine—maybe after an evening bath or when you wake up in the morning.

- When you visit your doctor, make sure he or she checks your feet, too. A foot inspection should be a part of every doctor's visit.

- Make sure your shoes fit properly. Poorly fitting shoes are an invitation to a callus or a blister. Measure your feet the next time you purchase shoes. Your feet may have changed (or your memory may have betrayed you) since the last time you measured.

- Wear running shoes or walking shoes. They're comfortable, lightweight, and soft.

- Wear padded socks that protect the bony parts of your feet. Some shoe or sporting-goods stores sell padded socks specially made for walking. They are luxuriously comfortable to wear, and they're good protection for your feet.

- Avoid hot soaks, heating pads, or electric blankets. Desensitized skin can burn.

- Avoid walking barefoot. This minimizes the risk of accidental cuts.

- If you get a callus or a blister, see your doctor. Stay away from over-the-counter corn or callus removers, because the chemicals in them are too harsh for a diabetic's skin. As Dr. Klombers advises, "If you're a diabetic, you should never cut corns or calluses, because the risk of injury and infection is too great."

- Build good circulation in your feet by walking or swimming, and by keeping your feet dry and warm.

DO GO EASY ON ALCOHOL   If you don't drink, good for you. If you are part of the majority who enjoy alcohol, diabetes doesn't mean you have to give it up. However, it does mean that you should exercise moderation. Most diabetics can tolerate an occasional beer, a glass of wine with dinner, or even a hard drink without much problem. But steady, daily consumption of alcohol—the so-called social drinking that most of us probably don't even notice—is not a good idea.

Alcohol lowers your blood sugar level. This can be a particular problem if you drink on an empty stomach. If food isn't in your stomach and you haven't eaten for some time, your body may have exhausted its reserves of glycogen (stored glucose). Since your body needs a steady supply of glucose at all times, it begins to convert fat or even protein to glucose, which it uses as fuel. (This is why starved people look thin; their bodies have begun to feed on their own fat and muscle.) But alcohol throws a wrench into this important glucose conversion process, shutting it down and leaving the body gasping for food. Blood sugar levels fall lower and lower. If they dip too low, you can develop hypoglycemia. The warning signs (see page 59) are legendary: faintness, weakness, anxiety, headache. You get confused, your vision gets blurred, your body movements become uncoordinated. At this point, unless you get some glucose into your system fast, you risk being paralyzed and winding up in a coma. You can imagine the potential disaster awaiting a diabetic who has a few drinks on an empty stomach and then climbs behind the wheel of a car.

If you drink, be thoughtful about it. Diabetics should avoid consuming sugar, and that includes sweet alcoholic drinks. Choose dry wine instead of sweet. Drink hard liquor on the rocks or with water or sparkling water instead of with soft drinks or fruit juices. Drink in moderation. And above all, don't drink on an empty stomach.

DON'T SMOKE   Smoking damages the inside lining of blood vessels. This hastens the growth of fatty deposits in your arteries, which can in turn lead to a stroke or heart attack. Since diabetics are already prone to atherosclerosis, diabetics who smoke are in double jeopardy.

But there's an even more important reason that smoking is dangerous for diabetics. Tobacco smoke contains carbon monoxide. When this poisonous gas enters the lungs, it clamps onto hemoglobin, a bloodstream compound responsible for carrying oxygen throughout the body. Carbon monoxide is selfish; it latches onto hemoglobin so fiercely that oxygen itself can't join up with hemoglobin. As a result, oxygen has no way of getting to the body's many tissues and cells. A smoker's blood may not contain enough life-giving oxygen to keep their extremities healthy. And if a smoker happens to suffer an infection far away from their lungs—in their feet, for example—their blood may not have enough oxygen to heal the infection. "Diabetics just shouldn't even think of smoking," diabetes expert Dr. W. James Howard of the Washington, DC, Medlantic Research Foundation told *Science News*.

So if you don't smoke now, celebrate your good fortune. If you do smoke, contact your local American Lung Association office for information on how black smokers can quit. And don't forget the American Cancer Society, which offers group sessions on how to stop smoking—and how to stay smoke-free. The sessions concentrate on weight control and stress management.

DO FIND HEALTHY WAYS OF MANAGING STRESS I don't need to tell you that this one has special significance for African-Americans. Anyone who wonders why the black community has such a high rate of stress-related health problems needs only consider the combined effects of poverty and racism, and the frustration and pent-up rage that accompany them.

But while stress has historically been linked to such health conditions as hypertension and heart disease, scientists now know diabetes has a stress connection as well. In fact, as Dr. Lois Jovanovic of the Manhattan (New York) Diabetes Self-Care Program told *Time* magazine, stress "can raise blood sugars higher than an ice cream sundae." Stress has such a striking impact that it can affect your blood sugar even though your diet, exercise, and medications may be just what the doctor prescribed for you.

What kind of stresses are we talking about? Feeling overloaded with responsibility. Having an argument with a loved one. Facing an unpleasant task. (In one study, a diabetic had to triple his insulin intake as the April 15 tax deadline drew near.) Some of the things that place demands on our bodies are normal biological functions, but they count as stresses nonetheless: menstruation; premenstrual syndrome (PMS); infection; injury; illness.

Coping with diabetes is stressful in itself. But in addition to the many emotional adjustments that newly diagnosed diabetics must make to accommodate the disease, diabetics face bias from others. "Unquestionably there has been and is discrimination against people with diabetes," says Dr. Leo Krall, president of the International Diabetes Federation, "just as there often is against anyone who is different." For example, when a group of English nursing schools were asked if they would accept diabetic nursing students, 111 schools said they would if the disease were completely controlled, 34 expressed strong reservations and suggested the women should pursue different careers, and 12 others said they would never accept any such applicants under any circumstances. When you consider the discrimination that faces these mostly white women—women whose race gives them certain privileges—it's disturbing to consider the barriers that confront persons of color. After all, our community has nowhere near the employment freedom that the white community has. Any discrimination against us because of an employer's inaccurate preconceptions about diabetes adds a bitter layer of disappointment and distress to our already difficult task of making ends meet.

Finally, getting decent health care for diabetes can be stressful. For example, 90 percent of poor diabetics have a doctor that they usually visit for care, according to a National Health Interview Survey. But only 70 percent of poor black diabetics have access to such a doctor. The same survey asked respondents if in the past year they had experienced problems getting health care because no care was available, they had no transportation, they didn't know where to go for care, the care was too expensive, or the hours at the health facility were inconvenient. While about 9 percent of nondiabetics reported having at least one of these problems, nearly twice as many diabetics—15 percent—did.

These many factors can combine to make life for black diabetics stressful indeed. The stress shows in many ways. Compared to black folks who are healthy, black diabetics typically suffer more psychiatric problems—from crying spells and loneliness to depression and even nervous breakdowns, according to the National Survey of Black Americans, a nationwide study funded by the National Institute of Mental Health. The irony, of course, is that the very stresses that produce these troubling emotional problems also worsen diabetes itself.

And that's why black folks need to seek out ways to manage anxiety and resolve worries. We need to find methods of handling difficult emotions and difficult situations in a way that affirms us instead of hurts us. Some of us find emotional equilibrium through exercise—daily walks, morning jogs, a midafternoon swim at the "Y." Some of my patients do yoga, others meditate, still others find their peace with a soothing, relaxing soak in the tub at the end of long day.

I'm convinced that these techniques can help black diabetics manage stress. At Duke University, Dr. Richard Surwit has helped Type 2 diabetics learn a technique called "progressive relaxation." The idea is simple, really. As you lie relaxed on your back, eyes closed, you tense your toes for a few seconds and then relax them. Then you do the same with your feet. Gradually you work your way to your face and head, patiently squeezing and relaxing all of the major muscle groups. Progressive relaxation is wonderfully calming to the spirit. And it's great for the body, too: once the diabetics had finished the relaxation training, they tolerated a dose of sugar better than did diabetics who had medication but no training.

DO WATCH YOUR WEIGHT Body weight and Type 2 diabetes are so intertwined that in many patients, losing weight eliminates the disease entirely. Now, no one says that losing weight is easy. It's not. The reasons we overeat are often complex and deeply imbedded in our psyche and even in our genes. Poverty plays a role. Black American men who are poor are slightly less likely to be fat than are men who live above the poverty line, but black women are nearly twice as likely compared to more affluent black women. Family habits, cultural expectations, stresses on the job and at home, loneliness and separation from loved ones—all these and more can prompt us to eat more food than our body needs. Certain illnesses can also cause obesity, among them thyroid conditions and disturbances of sex hormones in women. And fatness also seems to be inherited, at least in some families.

If you are thin and diabetes runs in your family, make a conscious effort to stay thin. Preventing obesity is a lot easier than trying to lose weight later on. If you are obese and you have diabetes, experts recommend essentially the same treatment as they do for other hefty people: eat a little less and exercise a little more. You might also consider some additional tools. Research suggests that psychotherapy is useful in weight loss, especially for people who were obese by the time they reached puberty. Diet counseling seems to be most effective for people whose obesity began at age twenty or older.

The key to success is gradual weight loss—no more than one or two pounds a week. I'll cover the specifics of good eating and exercise plans in Chapters 6 and 7.

STAYING ON TOP OF IT ALL

Doctors' visits, eye checkups, urine tests, blood pressure checks—it's all a lot to keep up with. Doctors lump these many keys to good health under the general heading of "compliance." If a patient does the things they're asked to do to stay healthy, they're in compliance with the doctor's advice.

As a rule, when it comes to diabetes the black community has a mediocre compliance record. Mind you, it's not always our fault. Most African-Americans live in the inner city, where health care is mostly dispensed from clinics. Diabetics at these settings have poorer compliance than patients who see private doctors, partly because the care at clinics is often subpar. I mentioned earlier the long waiting times, inconvenient clinic hours, overcrowded facilities, and callous staffs that, unfortunately, characterize many clinics. These have a tremendously negative impact on compliance by black diabetics, an effect by no means confined to the United States. A 1991 study of black Type 2 diabetics in South Africa found that no less than 65 percent failed to comply with their treatment program. Writing in the *South Africa Medical Journal*, the researchers who tracked the patients cited "inconvenient and inefficient clinics" and "patient dissatisfaction," along with such reasons as the unwanted side effects of medications. American critics who claim poor people and persons of color are sicker because we're too irresponsible or complacent to practice preventive care or even to keep our clinic appointments should take note: sick people are a sign of a sick health care system.

Having said that, I must also stress that every African-American with diabetes owes it to themselves and their loved ones to take complete charge of their health. If you have diabetes, you must be the first line of defense for your body. Only you can practice the healthy lifestyle that brings the disease under control. Your doctor cannot do it for you. As Duke psychologist Dr. Richard Surwit reminded *Psychology Today*, "Diabetes is perhaps the best example we have of a disease in which the patient's behavior is the key to the outcome."

Can the African-American community overcome its poor compliance record? We have no choice! No one can do it for us. Here are some ways to stay motivated and focused to do the things you need for good health:

FIND A DOCTOR WHO SEES LOTS OF DIABETES   Every doctor learns the basics of diabetes in medical school, but not everyone sees many patients with diabetes. Research shows that doctors who don't handle many cases of diabetes not only know less about it but are also less interested in the disease. And if your doctor isn't particularly interested in your condition, it's awfully hard for you to feel motivated to be healthy on your own. Find a doctor or a clinic with a reputation for seeing lots of diabetic patients. Chances are that's where you will find health care professionals who know the most about the disease and are most interested in it. That attitude rubs off on patients in the form of better motivation to get healthy and stay healthy.

FORGE A CONTRACT WITH YOUR DOCTOR   When many patients visit a doctor, they see the event as a one-way exchange. "Most of my patients basically want me to fix whatever ails them as fast as I can," reflects Dr. Ronald Shorr, a geriatrics specialist at the Vanderbilt University Medical Center. "I can talk all day about good health habits, but invariably they look at me and say, 'Just give me a pill, doc.'"

That doesn't work with diabetes. There's no magic pill. Instead, doctor and patient must work together. The doctor provides education, gives advice, dispenses medicine, and monitors how the patient is responding. The patient learns what they can about diabetes, establishes healthy habits, maintains those habits, and gives the doctor feedback on how the management of the disease is progressing. Together, doctor and patient forge a partnership.

Do you want to make a serious commitment to good health? Then ask your doctor to make a contract with you. Ask the doctor to spell out in writing a description of the goals the two of you want to achieve and what steps you need to take to accomplish those goals. Don't forget to include the things the doctor will do. Once you agree to the terms on the contract, both of you should sign it, just as you do any other contract. Health care contracts reinforce in both the patient and the doctor a strong commitment to good health.

MAKE SURE YOUR FAMILY FUNCTIONS WELL   Diabetics who live in dysfunctional families don't control their diabetes nearly as easily as those who live in healthy families. When researchers at Baylor College of Medicine in Houston studied the families of 385 low-income black, Hispanic, and white patients with Type 2 diabetes, they found that 92 percent of the patients who were controlling their diabetes well had families who shared decision-making, gave each other mutual support and caring, and were committed to devoting time to each other. In contrast, only 66 percent of the patients who had fair control of diabetes, and just 50 percent of patients who had poor control, had healthy families.

Dr. Lilia Cárdenas, the head of the research team, explained that it's much easier to work toward good health if you're in a healthy environment. "Since most of our patients required weight reduction, more than half were using insulin, and two-thirds of them had complications or...hypertension," Dr. Cárdenas said, "it is clear that they had a need for a nurturing environment that could help them comply with such complex prescribed treatments."

If your family doesn't function very well, then learning how to work together and be a healthier family might help you be a healthier diabetic. Find someone to talk to for guidance. This may be a family therapist, a social worker, a psychologist, a clergy member, or perhaps a respected elder.

MAKE GOOD HEALTH A HABIT   Have you ever been faced with a new responsibility that was so important that you weren't sure you could live up to the challenge? The first time you drove your family's car, weren't you nervous about having an accident? When you carried your newborn baby home from the hospital, didn't you wonder if you could be a good enough parent? These concerns are perfectly normal. They show that we feel a healthy sense of responsibility for our actions. Over time, as we drive the car more and more, and as we practice parenting day by day, we become surer of ourselves and our skills improve.

Daily practice is the key to managing diabetes, too. You may initially feel overwhelmed with your new responsibilities as a diabetic. There's a lot to remember, and there are lots of emotions to sort out. You may feel that controlling diabetes takes energy that you're not sure you can muster. But give it a try. Make diabetes care a part of your daily routine. Before long, you may fall into a habit of monitoring your blood sugar and planning your diet just as routinely as you comb your hair or brush your teeth. As one diabetic wrote, "Carrying an insulin kit, a blood sugar testing device and assorted snacks, and sticking to a regular schedule of eating, I have forgotten what it was like not to consider all of these details."

REMEMBER THE IMPORTANCE OF PREVENTION   They say a stitch in time saves nine. That may be trite, but I can tell you for a fact that when it comes to diabetes, truer words have never been spoken. Diabetes rewards people who make a beeline to their doctor when they feel bad, instead of putting off a visit, hoping they'll feel better. It rewards people who can summon the strength to make a small sacrifice today to feel healthy and avoid a larger problem tomorrow. It rewards people who faithfully follow their doctor's advice every day instead of waiting until they wake from a diabetic coma before they resolve to change their ways.

Medical science has made tremendous strides since I started seeing diabetes patients in 1950. Today even if a patient comes into my office in the advanced stages of diabetes, I can discuss tools that were hardly imaginable in earlier years. Back then, when a diabetic's pancreas was failing, about all we could do was put them on a good diet, give them insulin, and hope. Nowadays researchers are transplanting pancreas glands to give a diabetic a dramatically new life. Scientists have even invented a plastic pancreas that can be installed in place of the real thing.

These remarkable remedies don't come cheap, however. A pancreas transplant, for example, can cost in the neighborhood of $40,000. Medical treatments usually follow a simple rule: the longer you wait, the more they cost. It's easy and inexpensive to arrest a medical problem in the early stages. As time passes, it becomes more difficult and more costly. And sometimes, as with the blindness that can result from diabetic retinopathy, it becomes impossible.

That's why I advise my patients to think in terms of preventing the complications of diabetes instead of curing them. The tips in this chapter will start you in the right direction. Think of them as an appetizer. If you're ready to jump in with both feet, read on. Because I have a lot to share with you about three of the most important tools you can use to manage diabetes and stay healthy, whole, and happy. I like to call this multipronged strategy a "three-legged stool." You'll understand why in the next chapter.

WATCHING WHAT YOU EAT

In 1975 a twenty-four-year-old woman visited my office complaining of the recent onset of classic signs of diabetes: thirst, frequent urination, and weight loss despite a large intake of food. She was an intelligent high school graduate with an addiction to junk foods and rich desserts. After several consultations with me and a dietician, she gave up her junk foods and readily accepted insulin therapy. Today she takes insulin each day and is the proud owner of an exercise bicycle. Best of all, although she has mild nerve damage, she has no kidney impairment and no eye problems. Here is a young woman who has diabetes but who likes to go out with friends and finds that a diabetic diet fits in with most restaurant menus. Her diet has not compromised her social life or her lifestyle.

Millions of people manage to control their diabetes and go on to lead healthy, enriching lives. No two of them are alike. Some diabetics are twelve years old, others eighty-two. Some are unemployed, others head corporations. Some diabetics are even famous. Singer Ella Fitzgerald controls her diabetes successfully.

But despite their differences, there's one thing that every successful diabetic has in common. They have introduced three essential elements to their daily lives—good food, moderate exercise, and careful medication. These are the three keys to making sure your blood sugar level stays in the safe zone—not too high, not too low.

Diabetes doesn't prevent you from enjoying life to the very fullest. If you're an athlete, you can still play sports. (Baseball great Jackie Robinson had diabetes.) If you're a natural comedian, you can still be the life of the party. (Actress Nell Carter has diabetes.) But you must remember these three items—food, exercise, and medication. And because these important aspects of life have different effects on your blood sugar, you must find a way to bring them into balance.

One of the best ways to imagine this balancing act is to picture your health as a stool supported by three legs. One leg is diet, the second is exercise, and the third is medication. If one leg is weak, the stool will be shaky. If all of them are weak, it will come crashing to the floor quicker than you can say "insulin." On the other hand, if the legs are strong, the stool will have a firm foundation. And as long as each leg stays strong, the stool will stay strong, too.

That's exactly what I see in my diabetic patients. Patients who watch what they eat but don't take the time to exercise and aren't careful about their medication aren't as healthy as they could be. Unfortunately, those who give up on all three—and eat poorly, live a sedentary life, and neglect their medication entirely—invite disaster, and frequently get it. Having diabetes and enjoying life in good, sound health is entirely possible, but it takes a commitment to keep each of the three legs of the stool good and solid.

Let's spend some time taking a look at the first leg—your new diet.

YOU ARE WHAT YOU EAT

For years, the diabetic diet had one prominent feature. If you asked anyone with diabetes what the thrust of managing their diet was, they would tell you, "I can't eat sugar." That's not true any more. Small amounts of sugar are fine when they are eaten as part of a meal. This may strike you as a revolutionary idea, especially if, like many African-Americans, you grew up believing the popular (but mistaken) advice that diabetes was *caused* by too much sugar. But the old approach of managing diabetes solely by controlling sugar intake is out. What's in is placing fiber and carbohydrates front and center and giving protein a back seat.

Here are the goals of a good diabetic diet that we'll cover in this chapter:

1. Because diabetes carries a risk of damage to arteries, the most beneficial diet is *low in saturated fat and cholesterol.*

2. Because high blood glucose damages tissues, foods that help normalize blood glucose levels should be plentiful. That means *generous fiber* and *limited sugar.*

3. Because excess body fat causes insulin resistance and high blood glucose, *calories should be appropriate for weight loss.*

4. Because too much protein puts a strain on the kidneys, and most of us eat more protein than we need anyway, *protein should be eaten in moderation.*

5. Because insulin takes effect at different times, every effort should be made to *maintain a regular schedule for eating.*

These are the same goals that nutritionists recommend for people who don't have diabetes. The difference is that we are trying to use dietary choices to control specific symptoms. These food choices benefit more people than just you. As a diabetic, once you change your diet to promote your health, the whole household eats better.

Table 1 shows what these changes actually mean in a recommended diet.

I find it easier to follow recommendations if I understand the basis for them. So the remainder of this chapter expands on the suggestions in Table 1.

TABLE 1   Foods for Controlling Symptoms and Long-term
Complications of Diabetes

Goal	Strategy	Examples	Amount
Maintain normal blood glucose	Eat high-fiber foods	Dried peas and beans Vegetables Oatmeal, whole grain breads & cereals	3–5 servings a day
	Limit sugars	Table sugar Fruit juices Whole fruits Fructose	1 tsp/meal 4 oz/meal 3–5/day As desired
	Limit alcohol	Beer, wine, liquor	None or 1/day
	Use sugar substitutes	Aspartame, saccharin Sorbitol, mannitol hydrogenated starch hydrolysate (HSH)	As desired less than 5 servings a day
Maintain healthy body weight	Limit total fat	Margarine, salad dressing, oil, mayonnaise	6–7 tsp/day
		Fatty meats, whole milk, cheese	Avoid
		Lean meats, lowfat cheese, 1% fat milk	Use daily
	Limit total calories	Vegetables, cereals, breads, beans, pasta, lean poultry, fish, meat, lowfat milk and milk products, fruit	Moderate portions
Prevent artery damage	Limit total fat	(Same as above)	
	Limit saturated fat	(Same as above)	
	Limit cholesterol	Eggs Organ meats	4 per week Avoid

HOW FOOD AFFECTS
BLOOD GLUCOSE LEVELS

Your level of blood glucose is directly influenced by the amount and kind of carbohydrates in your diet. Table 2 gives examples of sources of carbohydrates.

As you may remember from Chapter 1, carbohydrates are the

TABLE 2 Sources of Carbohydrates

Type	Name	Found in
Simple sugar	Glucose	Fruits, juices, syrup, small amounts in vegetables
	Fructose	Fruits, corn, other sugar syrups
	Sucrose	Fruits, syrup, small amounts in vegetables, table sugar, sweetened foods, beverages
	Lactose	Milk, yogurt, cheese
	Dextrose	Small amounts in fruits and vegetables, also added to foods in small amounts
Complex sugar	Starch	Beans, peas, wheat, rice, oats, corn, barley, root vegetables (potatoes, yams, turnips), foods made from these (bread, crackers, pasta, etc.)
Fiber	Cellulose, hemicellulose pectin, gum, lignin	All plants, skins and hulls of fruits, grains, vegetables (see Table 3 for details)

body's principal fuel. Calories are a measure of just how much fuel a food contains. All carbohydrates contain four calories per gram.

There are several types of carbohydrates. Simple carbohydrates, also called simple sugars, are made of either one molecule of sugar or two molecules of sugar attached to each other. Glucose, the body's basic fuel, is a one-molecule simple carbohydrate. So is fructose, or fruit sugar. On the other hand, sucrose, or table sugar, is a two-molecule simple carbohydrate. Lactose, a sugar found in milk, is a two-molecule carbohydrate as well.

If you eat a simple carbohydrate with no other food, the sugar moves from the intestines to the bloodstream very quickly. As a result, foods that contain lots of simple sugars often raise blood glucose levels dramatically. Sometimes that can be a lifesaver for a person with diabetes. If you've exercised too vigorously on an empty stomach, taken insulin or diabetes medication without eating, or taken too much insulin or diabetes medication altogether, your blood sugar may dip too low. In this case, the rapid absorption of sugars in fruit juice or candy can restore blood sugar levels to normal. But if your blood sugar level is moderate to begin with, simple carbohydrates can raise it above the safe range. That's why the American Diabetes Association recommends that no more than 10 percent of a diabetic's total calories should come from simple carbohydrates.

For *complex* carbohydrates, the advice is just the opposite. People with diabetes should make complex carbohydrates an important part of each day's diet. Complex carbohydrates are composed of the same basic sugars that make up simple carbohydrates. But research shows that a diet high in complex carbohydrates—starch and fiber—may promote healthy blood glucose levels.

If simple carbohydrates (sugar) and complex carbohydrates (starch and fiber) contain the same building blocks, why are complex carbohydrates so much better for us? The reason is the building blocks are arranged differently. The sugar molecules in simple carbohydrates are short and easy for the body to digest. On the other hand, the sugar molecules in complex carbohydrates are long and must be broken apart by enzymes in the small intestine before the body can get at the sugars within.

Think of simple carbohydrates as a single Lifesaver® candy. Pop it in your mouth and you get instant gratification. Complex carbohydrates are like a *case* of Lifesavers®. To enjoy one candy, you must break open a cardboard box, unwrap a cellophane liner, tear apart a paper sleeve, and peel open a foil wrapper. It takes time before the candy makes it to your mouth. Similarly, it takes time for your body's digestive enzymes to break down complex carbohydrates like starches into simple sugars. Because the sugars are released into the bloodstream gradually, these complex carbohydrates don't cause the sharp rise in blood glucose levels that simple carbohydrates do. (Make sure you understand this is just an example of how starches differ from sugars and that you should not consider eating a case of Lifesavers®—even slowly.)

Fiber reacts still differently. There are several kinds of fiber (Table 3), but the two main forms are water-soluble and water-insoluble. What sets all fiber apart from other carbohydrates is that our digestive tract can't break it down at all into simple carbohydrates. Unlike termites or cows, people lack the stomach enzymes for this task.

TABLE 3 Fiber in Foods

Kind of fiber	Where it's found	What it does
Water-Soluble		
Gums and mucilage	Beans, peas, seeds, bran, oats, many vegetables	Forms a gel, slows absorption of glucose, softens stool, lowers blood cholesterol
Pectin	Apples, berries, citrus fruits; many fruits, some vegetables	(Same as above)
Water-Insoluble		
Cellulose	All plants; skins, hulls and seed coats of fruits, vegetables, grains and beans	Bulks stool, relieves constipation (notably wheat bran); reduces insulin requirement
Hemicellulose	(Same as above)	(Same as above)
Lignin (not a carbo-hydrate)	Woody texture of vegetables, fruits	(Same as above)

Nonetheless, fiber is extremely valuable. Water-soluble fiber (gums and pectin) absorbs water as it travels through the intestine. That water combines with the gum or pectin to form a gel that surrounds the food that's being digested. This means that digestive enzymes must first penetrate the gel before they can reach the food. And that slows the rate of digestion, thereby causing a slower, gentler, more sustained passage of glucose into the bloodstream. That's why an apple (which is sweet but rich in fiber) causes a less dramatic surge of blood sugar than does a candy bar (which is rich in simple sugar but contains little fiber). Water-soluble fiber also lowers cholesterol levels in your blood, which is why oat bran and other fiber-rich foods such as beans are recommended to help prevent heart disease.

Water-insoluble fiber (the chewy portion of edible plants) passes through the digestive tract untouched. But in so doing, it reduces the amount of insulin your body needs to process glucose. It also sweeps the intestines clean and gives beneficial bulk to your stool. Diets rich in water-insoluble fiber offer protection from cancer of the bowel.

Foods high in soluble fiber—dried peas, beans, apples—are nearly ideal for causing the lowest rise in blood glucose. Traditional African-American cooking offers a number of bean-based dishes, from the blackeye peas of Hoppin' John to savory succotash to red beans and rice. Ideally, your diet should include a host of peas and beans. Serve them twice a day in main dishes, side dishes, and in salads.

All in all, you should obtain 50 to 60 percent of your total calories from carbohydrates, and you should consume at least forty grams of fiber each day. Again, no more than 10 percent of your total calories should come from simple sugars, making starches your major source of carbohydrates. This may take some time to work up to, but it should improve your blood glucose levels substantially.

Some people wonder if the fiber supplements you can purchase in pharmacies and supermarkets can lower glucose as well as natural fiber from food does. They may not. For best results, I recommend sticking with real food.

To repeat, these recommendations to eat plenty of carbohydrates may seem like sacrilege to an older diabetic. Years ago, doctors advised diabetics to restrict carbohydrates but to eat plenty of fat and protein. So diabetics placed careful limits on bread, rice, and sweets, and chowed down on bacon, luncheon meats, cheeses, and other fatty meaty proteins. Nowadays, we know that many of the health risks in diabetes are caused by high-fat diets, and probably high-protein diets as well. So today's advice is the polar opposite of what it was fifteen or twenty years ago.

Now that nutritionists have opened the door—slightly—to simple sugars for diabetics, you may find yourself mulling over questions about sweeteners:

What are "nonnutritive sweeteners," and are they safe?

Nonnutritive sweeteners are sugar substitutes, and they are fine to include in your food choices. They are called nonnutritive because they contain few or no calories. Aspartame, saccharin, and asulfame-K are all part of this family. These sweeteners often contain dextrose or maltodextrin, but these carbohydrates, added as bulking agents, occur in insignificant amounts.

Then what are "nutritive sweeteners?"

Nutritive sweeteners supply calories. Examples include sugar, corn syrup (also called "corn sweetener" on food labels), honey, fruit juice, or fructose. Many food packagers that label their baked goods and beverages "sugar-free" use one of these sweeteners. Of the lot, fructose is the best sweetener for diabetics because it has a very small effect on blood glucose levels. The drawback with fructose is that it is very expensive as crystals, and its sweetening power varies from use to use. It is wonderful in cold mixtures or when blended with fruits. In hot drinks or baked items, its sweetness is quite diminished. Even so, keep your fructose intake rather low.

Other nutritive sweeteners include sorbitol, mannitol, xylitol, and hydrogenated starch hydrolysate (HSH). These are sometimes found in candies, chewing gum, and other products that are typically labeled "sugar-free" but not "low-calorie." They are fine in small amounts. However, more than three or four packs of sorbitol-sweetened gum or mints may cause diarrhea.

Are there ways to sweeten without using a sweetener at all?

Some people find that cinnamon and nutmeg impart a subtle sweetness to many foods and beverages.

Do all sweeteners count against my overall carbohydrate total for a given day?

Yes. If a sweetener is a carbohydrate (see Table 2), it must be considered in your overall carbohydrate intake. I'll discuss this in greater detail in an upcoming section on meal planning.

Protein

Protein is an important part of everyone's diet. Protein is used to build all cells, hormones, and enzymes, and it makes up the bulk of your muscles, skin, hair, and blood cells. If you can picture muscle or skin as a brick house, protein forms the brick. Our bodies manufacture these bricks from twenty-two different amino acids. Of the twenty-two, the body can produce fourteen on its own. These are called *nonessential amino acids*, because it's not essential to eat them. The other eight must be supplied by our food. These are called *essential amino acids*.

Dietary protein comes from many sources. Foods that contain all of the eight essential amino acids (plus varying amounts of nonessential amino acids) are called *complete proteins*. Foods that contain some but not all of the essential amino acids (plus some nonessential amino acids) are called *incomplete proteins* (Table 4).

The American diet has always emphasized complete proteins. Turkeys and hams are the centerpiece of holiday gatherings, eggs and bacon form the classic American breakfast, and when surveys ask for our all-around favorite foods, we name hamburgers—and more recently pizza.

But it is very easy to get complete protein from a diet in which flesh, milk products, and eggs are limited or absent. Combining legumes (beans and peas) and grains ensures that we get the eight essential amino acids. This is the essence of how vegetarians select meals that are both delicious and nutritionally complete. Consider traditional favorites such as peas and rice, beans and cornbread, and even thinly spread peanut butter and bread. All of these are appropriate for diabetes because they are 1) a complete protein

TABLE 4 Sources of Protein

Type of protein	Food sources	Advantages	Disadvantages
Complete	Flesh: fish, poultry, red meat, organ meat	High iron	Unless lean, may be high in cholesterol High in fat High in saturated fat
	Milk, yogurt, cheese	High calcium	May be high in fat High in saturated fat
	Eggs		High cholesterol
	Soybeans	High fiber	
Incomplete	Legumes: beans, peas	High fiber Good iron	No cholesterol
	Peanut butter	(Same)	May be high in fat
	Grains: wheat, rice, oats, barley, corn	(Same as above)	
	Nuts and seeds	(Same as above)	
	Vegetables	Fair iron	

with 2) complex carbohydrates that are 3) high in fiber, 4) low in fat, and 5) cholesterol-free.

Plant proteins may have helped our ancestors avoid diabetes. Throughout the African continent, there is little diabetes in cultures that still maintain their traditional way of life. That lifestyle includes a diet that contains plenty of whole grains, dried beans and peas, and starchy and green vegetables—but remarkably little meat. In Arizona, home of the Pima tribe where diabetes runs rampant, researchers have found that when healthy volunteers consume dishes containing starchy foods that were once the mainstay of the Pimas—lima beans, corn, acorns, mesquite pods—their carbohydrate digestion slows down and their insulin and blood glucose levels are much lower than after eating conventional starches like potatoes and bread. There may be some real advantages to sticking with the diet that evolution has prepared our bodies to use.

Here's another good reason to eat more protein from plant foods: You are more likely to get only as much protein as you need without getting an excess amount. Nutritionists say the typical American diet contains over one-hundred grams of protein a day. We need only half of that amount (45 grams of protein for women and 56 grams of protein for men).

When you eat protein from plant foods you get less protein to the "bite" than you do with animal protein foods (such as meat). A high-protein diet gives the kidneys extra work. It may, in fact, increase some peoples' susceptibility to kidney damage and failure. Diabetes already heightens the risk of kidney damage. So, it's best to eat only as much protein as you need. That means, aim for as much plant protein as possible. It delivers protein as well as important complex carbohydrates. If you eat animal protein, choose items that are low in total fat and saturated fat.

Fat

As nutrients go, fat is pretty deceptive. On the one hand, it has plenty of good points. Fats absorb flavors extremely well, and they add magnificent flavor to foods. (People who have tasted experimentally defatted chicken say it has so little flavor that they couldn't tell what kind of meat it was.) Fat takes a long time to be digested, so a fatty meal helps us feel full longer by remaining in the stomach. Fat is also an important nutrient. It stores calories during times when we consume more calories than we can immediately burn; it also enhances the absorption of fat-soluble vitamins (A, D, E, and K) from the intestines.

Where's the deception? Well for starters, over half of the fat in our national diet is hidden. It's not the butter that sits in plain view on the butter dish or the cooking oil that we pour into a skillet. It's the fat in pastries and convenience foods and nuts and meat and milk—fat we can't really see.

The ultimate deception, of course, is that something so inviting can be so dangerous. Eating too much fat has been linked to an increased risk of heart disease, atherosclerosis, and obesity, not to mention diabetes. The fact that much of the fat that we eat is hidden cannot obscure the reality that we bring these problems on ourselves: when it comes to fat, most of us are like children in a candy store. "In the standard American diet, the fat in foods has taken a position all out of proportion to its necessary role," writes Laurel Robertson, author of *Laurel's Kitchen: A Handbook of Vegetarian Cookery and Nutrition* (New York: Bantam Books, 1982). Most Americans receive around 40 percent of their calories from fat, this despite the fact that our bodies need relatively little fat to live and thrive. That's significantly more than the 30 percent that nutritionists recommend.

The amount of fat that you eat, and the type of fat it is, can raise or lower your level of blood cholesterol, especially LDL (low-density lipoprotein) cholesterol, a type of cholesterol that leads to atherosclerosis and heart disease. If you have diabetes, you, like all Americans, should get very few of your total calories—no more than 30 percent—from fat. Of that 30 percent, less than one third should come from saturated fat—the fat that elevates LDL cholesterol levels. Another third or less of daily fat should come from polyunsaturated fat. The final third or more should come from monounsaturated fats. Table 5 shows which types of fats appear in which foods.

To achieve your goal of no more than 30 percent of fat in your diet, try to eat no more than fifty to sixty-five grams of fat each day. If

TABLE 5 Predominant Types of Fats in Foods

Polyunsaturated	Moderate Amounts of Polyunsaturated	Monounsaturated	Saturated
Safflower oil	Soybean oil	Olive oil	Beef fat/suet
Walnut oil	Mayonnaise	Canola oil	Butter fat
Sunflower oil	Salad dressing	Rapeseed oil	Lamb fat
Corn oil	Tub margarine	Peanut oil	Pork fat/lard
Sunflower seeds		Stick margarine	Canned shortening
		Avocado	Meat drippings
		Cashews	
		Peanuts	
		Pecans	

Poultry and fish have approximately equal amounts of polyunsaturated, monounsaturated, and saturated fats.

Note: Only spreads, cooking fats, and dressings that contain three or more grams of fat per teaspoon are listed here. Spreads that are fat-free or very low in fat, having less than one gram of fat per teaspoon, are not listed.

you develop the habit of scanning food labels, you will find that many manufacturers list the amount—and the type—of fat in each serving.

One note on fish oil. You may have heard of the benefits of something called omega-3 fatty acids. These are oils contained in fish that live in cold ocean depths—tuna, salmon, sardines, herring, and mackerel. Omega-3's are thought to help protect the body against cardiovascular disease, rheumatoid arthritis, psoriasis—and yes, diabetes. At least two national health organizations, the American Heart Association and the American Dietetic Association, recommend eating fish two or three times a week. I think that's good advice, but avoid large amounts of omega-3 oil, including fish oil capsules, because it may raise your blood glucose level.

All fats, whether from animals or plants, contain nine calories per gram.

HOW TO PLAN YOUR MEALS

Three squares is the name of the game. A missed meal, even a late meal, can have serious consequences, particularly if you take insulin. Headache, dizziness, sweating, irritability, and the more serious consequences of low blood sugar can be avoided by planning morning, midday, and evening meals. Most people also find that a couple of snacks, included in the calorie goal, will make the day smoother.

When you have diabetes, you need to time your meals for a point in the day when insulin activity, whether injected or stimulated by pills, is at its peak. Since carbohydrates are the most important influence on blood sugar levels, which in turn are linked to your need for insulin, here's a rule of thumb when planning your daily carbohydrate intake. Of your total carbohydrates you should eat:

- 30 percent in the morning meal
- 30 percent in the midday meal
- 10 percent in snacks
- 30 percent in the evening meal.

You can find out whether a certain meal matches the available insulin by checking your blood glucose levels during the day, particularly before meals. Some people find that five or six small meals a day are more helpful than three meals in managing their blood glucose levels.

To make meal planning easy, use "exchange lists" developed by the American Diabetes Association and the American Dietetic Association (Table 6). If you're trying to lose weight, you're in luck; many weight-loss programs adapt these same lists to help their patrons control their calories.

Exchange lists are designed around four points:

1. *Nutrient similarity.* Foods composed of essentially the same amount and kind of nutrients (carbohydrate, protein, fat) are included in the same exchange list. For example, all vegetables are grouped together, and all starchy foods are listed together.

There are six exchanges or lists:

- Starch or bread
- Meat and meat alternatives
- Vegetable
- Fruit

- Milk
- Fat

2. *Uniform amounts of nutrients.* By controlling portion sizes, each food on any given list provides the same amount of calories, carbohydrate, protein, and fat. For example (from the Starch/Bread exchange list), three fourths of a cup of corn flakes is equivalent to one third of a cup of rice, one slice of bread, or three fourths of an ounce of pretzels. By following these lists, you can plan a meal calling for two portions of starch by selecting any two items on the starch/bread exchange list (using the portions given) or by doubling any one item.

In fact, you can plan an entire day's menu by building your meals around the nutrients in each exchange list:

EXCHANGE LIST	CARBOHYDRATE (grams)	PROTEIN (grams)	FAT (grams)	CALORIES
Starch/bread	15	3	trace	80
Meat and meat alternate				
Lean	0	7	3	55
Medium fat	0	7	5	75
High fat	0	7	8	100
Vegetable	5	2	0	25
Fruit	15	0	0	60
Milk				
Skim/very lowfat	12	8	trace	90
Lowfat	12	8	5	120
Whole milk	12	8	8	150
Fat	0	0	5	45

3. *Overall balance.* By drafting a basic daily menu, you can swap or exchange foods within lists and enjoy variety and dietary balance every day.

4. *Free or unlimited foods.* Many salad vegetables, herbs, non-

---

TABLE 6 Exchange Lists

C = cup; t = teaspoon; T = tablespoon

1. STARCH/BREAD EXCHANGES: Each item on this list contains 15 grams of carbohydrate, 3 grams of protein, a trace of fat, and 80 calories. One exchange is equal to any of the following items:

Cereals/Grains/Pasta

Bran cereals, concentrated	⅓ C
Bran cereals, flaked (such as Bran Buds, All Bran)	½ C
Bulgur	½ C
Cooked cereals	½ C
Cornmeal (dry)	2½ T
Grape Nuts	3 T
Grits (cooked)	½ C
Other ready-to-eat unsweetened cereals	¾ C
Pasta (cooked)	½ C
Puffed cereal	1½ C
Rice, white or brown (cooked)	⅓ C
Shredded wheat	½ C
Wheat germ	3 T

Dried Beans/Peas/Lentils

Beans and peas (cooked) (such as kidney, white, split, blackeye)	⅓ C
Lentils	⅓ C
Baked beans	¼ C

Starchy Vegetables

Corn	½ C
Corn on cob, 6" long	1
Lima beans	½ C
Peas, green (canned or frozen)	½ C
Plantain	½ C
Potato, baked, 1 small	(3 oz)
Potato, mashed	½ C
Squash, winter (acorn, butternut)	¾ C
Yam, sweet potato, plain	⅓ C

Bread

Bagel	½ (1 oz)
Bread sticks, crisps, 4" long x ½"	2 (⅔ oz)
Croutons, lowfat	1 C
English muffin	½
Frankfurter or hamburger bun	½ (1 oz)
Pita, 6" across	½
Plain roll, small	1 (1 oz)
Raisin, unfrosted	1 slice (1 oz)
Rye, pumpernickel	1 slice (1 oz)
Tortilla, 6" across	1
White (including French, Italian)	1 slice (1 oz)
Whole wheat	1 slice (1 oz)

Crackers/Snacks

Animal crackers	8
Graham crackers, 2½" square	3
Matzoh	¾ oz
Melba toast	5 slices
Oyster crackers	24
Popcorn (popped, no fat added)	3 C
Pretzels	¾ oz
Rye crisps, 2" x 3½"	4
Saltine-type crackers	6
Whole wheat crackers, 2–4 slices (¾ oz) no fat added (crisps, breads, such as Finn, Kavli, Wasa)	

Starchy Foods Prepared With Fat
(Count as 1 starch/bread serving plus 1 fat serving)

Biscuit, 2½" across	1

Chow mein noodles	½ C
Corn bread, 2" cube	1 (2 oz)
Cracker, round butter type	6
French fried potatoes, 10 (1½ oz) 2" to 3½" long	
Muffin, plain, small	1

Pancake, 4" across	2
Stuffing, bread (prepared)	¼ C
Taco shell, 6" across	2
Waffle, 4½" square	1
Whole wheat, fat added (such as Triscuits)	4–6 (1 oz)

2. MEAT EXCHANGES

A. LEAN MEAT AND SUBSTITUTES: Each item on this list contains 7 grams of protein, 3 grams of fat, and 55 calories. One exchange is equal to any one of the following items:

Beef

USDA Good or Choice grades of lean beef, such as round, sirloin and flank steak; tenderloin; and chipped beef	1 oz

Pork

Lean pork, such as fresh ham; canned, cured or boiled ham, Canadian bacon, tenderloin	1 oz

Veal

All cuts are lean except for veal cutlets (ground or cubed). Examples of lean veal are chops and roasts	1 oz

Poultry

Chicken, turkey, Cornish hen (without skin)	1 oz

Fish

All fresh and frozen fish	1 oz
Crab, lobster, scallops, shrimp, clams (fresh or canned in water)	2 oz
Oysters	6 med
Tuna (canned in water)	¼ C
Herring (uncreamed or smoked)	1 oz
Sardines (canned)	2 med

Wild game

Venison, rabbit, squirrel	1 oz
Pheasant, duck, goose (without skin)	1 oz

Cheese

Any cottage cheese	¼ C

Grated Parmesan	2 T
Diet cheeses (with less than 55 calories per ounce)	1 oz

Other

95% fat-free luncheon meat	1 oz
Egg whites	3 whites
Egg substitutes with less than 55 calories per 1/4 C	¼ C

B. MEDIUM-FAT MEAT AND SUBSTITUTES: Each item on this list contains 7 grams of protein, 5 grams of fat, and 75 calories. One exchange is equal to any one of the following items:

Beef	1 oz
Most beef products fall into this category. Examples are: all ground beef, roast (rib, chuck, rump), steak (cubed, Porterhouse, T-bone), meatloaf	
Pork	1 oz
Most pork products fall into this category. Examples are: chops, loin roast, Boston butt, cutlets	
Lamb	1 oz
Most lamb products fall into this category. Examples are: chops, leg, and roast	
Poultry	1 oz
Chicken (with skin), domestic duck or goose (well-drained of fat), ground turkey	

Fish

Tuna (canned in oil and drained)	¼ C
Salmon (canned)	¼ C

Cheese

Skim or part-skim milk cheeses, such as: Ricotta	¼ C

continued on page 94

Mozzarella	1 oz
Diet cheeses	1 oz
(with 56–80 calories per ounce)	

Other

86% fat-free luncheon meat	1 oz
Egg (high in cholesterol, limit to 3 per week)	1
Egg substitutes with 56–80 calories per ¼ C	¼ C
Tofu (2½" x 2¾" x 1")	1
Liver, heart, kidney, sweetbreads (high in cholesterol)	1 oz

C. HIGH-FAT MEATS AND SUBSTITUTES: Each item on this list contains 7 grams protein, 8 grams fat, and 100 calories. Remember—these items are high in saturated fat, cholesterol, and calories, and should be used only three (3) times per week. One exchange is equal to any one of the following items:

Beef

Most USDA Prime cuts of beef, such as ribs, corned beef	1 oz
Pork	1 oz

Spareribs, ground pork, pork sausage (patty or link)	

Lamb

Patties (ground lamb)	1 oz

Fish

Any fried fish product	1 oz

Cheese

All regular cheeses, such as American, Blue, Cheddar, Monterey, Swiss	1 oz

Other

Luncheon meat, such as bologna, salami, pimento loaf	1 oz
Sausage, such as Polish, Italian	1 oz
Knockwurst, smoked	1 oz
Bratwurst	1 oz
Peanut butter (contains unsaturated fat)	1 T

Count as one high-fat meat plus one fat exchange:

Frankfurter (beef, pork or combination)	1 frank

---

3. VEGETABLE EXCHANGES: Each vegetable serving on this list contains 5 grams of carbohydrate, 2 grams of protein, and 25 calories. One exchange is ½ cup of cooked vegetables or ½ cup of vegetable juice or 1 cup of raw vegetables.

Artichoke (½ medium)	Eggplant	Rutabaga
Asparagus	Greens (collard, mustard, turnip)	Sauerkraut
Beans (green, wax, Italian)		Spinach, cooked
Bean sprouts	Kohlrabi	Summer squash (crookneck)
Beets	Leeks	
Broccoli	Mushrooms, cooked	Tomato (one large)
Brussels sprouts	Okra	Tomato/vegetable juice
Cabbage	Onions	Turnips
Carrots	Pea pods	Water chestnuts
Cauliflower	Peppers (green)	Zucchini, cooked

4. FRUIT EXCHANGES: Each item on this list contains 15 grams of carbohydrate and 60 calories. One exchange is equal to any one of the following items:

FRESH, FROZEN, OR UNSWEETENED CANNED FRUIT			
Apple (raw, 2" across)	1
Applesauce (unsweetened)	¹/₂ C
Apricots (medium, raw)	4
Apricots (canned)	¹/₂ C or 4 halves
Banana (9" long)	¹/₂
Blackberries (raw)	³/₄ C
Cantaloupe (5" across)	¹/₃
Cubes	1 C
Cherries (large, raw)	12
Cherries (canned)	¹/₂ C
Figs (raw, 2" across)	2
Fruit cocktail (canned)	¹/₂ C
Grapefruit (medium)	¹/₂
Grapefruit (segments)	³/₄ C
Grapes (small)	15
Honeydew melon (medium)	¹/₈
Cubes	1 C
Kiwi (large)	1
Mandarin oranges	³/₄ C
Mango (small)	¹/₂
Nectarine (1¹/₂" across)	1
Orange (2¹/₂" across)	1
Papaya	1 C
Peach (2³/₄" across)	1
Peaches (canned)	¹/₂ C or 2 halves

Pear	¹/₂ large or 1 small
Pears (canned)	¹/₂ C or 2 halves
Persimmon (medium)	2
Pineapple (raw)	³/₄ C
Pineapple (canned)	¹/₃ C
Plum (raw, 2" across)	2
Pomegranate	1/2
Raspberries (raw)	1 C
Strawberries (raw, whole)	1¹/₄ C
Tangerine (2¹/₂" across)	2
Watermelon (cubes)	1¹/₄ C

DRIED FRUIT

Apples	4 rings
Apricots	7 halves
Dates (medium)	2¹/₂
Figs	1¹/₂
Prunes (medium)	3
Raisins	2 T

FRUIT JUICE

Apple juice/cider	¹/₂ C
Cranberry juice cocktail	¹/₃ C
Grapefruit juice	¹/₂ C
Grape juice	¹/₃ C
Orange juice	¹/₂ C
Pineapple juice	¹/₂ C
Prune juice	¹/₃ C

5. MILK EXCHANGES

SKIM AND VERY LOWFAT MILK: Each item on this list contains 12 grams of carbohydrate, 8 grams of protein, a trace of fat, and 90 calories. One exchange is equal to any one of the following items:

Skim milk	1 C
1/2% milk	1 C
1% milk	1 C
Lowfat buttermilk	1 C

Evaporated skim milk	¹/₂ C
Dry nonfat milk	¹/₃ C
Plain nonfat yogurt	8 oz

LOWFAT MILK: Each item on this list contains 12 grams of carbohydrate, 8 grams of protein, 5 grams of fat, and 120 calories. One exchange is equal to one of the following items:

2% milk	1 C

continued on page 96

Plain lowfat yogurt   8 oz
(with added nonfat milk solids)

WHOLE MILK: Each item on this list contains 12 grams of carbohydrate, 8 grams of protein, 8 grams of fat, and 150 calories.

One exchange is equal to any one of the following items:

Whole milk	1 C
Evaporated whole milk	½ C
Whole plain yogurt	8 oz

6. FAT EXCHANGES: Each item on this list contains 5 grams of fat and 45 calories. One exchange is equal to any one of the following items:

UNSATURATED

Avocado	⅛ medium
Margarine	1 t
Margarine, diet	1 T
Mayonnaise	1 t
Mayonnaise, reduced-calorie	1 T
Nuts and seeds:	
Almonds, dry-roasted	6 whole
Cashews, dry-roasted	1 T
Pecans	2 whole
Peanuts	20 small or 10 large
Walnuts	2 whole
Other nuts	1 T
Seeds, pine nuts, sunflower (without shells)	1 T
Pumpkin seeds	2 t
Oil (corn, cottonseed, safflower, soybean, sunflower, olive, peanut)	1 t

Olives	10 small or 5 large
Salad dressing, mayonnaise-type	2 t
Salad dressing, mayonnaise-type, reduced-calorie	1 T
Salad dressing, all varieties	1 T
Salad dressing, reduced-calorie	2 T

SATURATED

Butter	1 t
Bacon	1 slice
Chitterlings	½ oz
Coconut, shredded	2 T
Coffee whitener, liquid	2 T
Coffee whitener, powder	4 T
Cream (light, coffee, table)	2 T
Cream, sour	2 T
Cream, heavy whipping	1 T
Cream cheese	1 T
Salt pork	¼ oz

FREE FOODS: A free food is any food or drink that contains less than 20 calories per serving. You can eat as much as you want of those items that have no serving size specified. You may eat two or three servings per day of those items that have a specific serving size. Be sure to spread them out through the day.

DRINKS

Bouillon or broth without fat

Bouillon, low-sodium

Carbonated drinks, sugar-free

Carbonated water

Club soda

Cocoa powder, unsweetened (1 T)

Coffee/tea

Drink mixes, sugar-free

Tonic water, sugar-free

NON-STICK PAN SPRAY

FRUIT

Cranberries, unsweetened (½ C)

Rhubarb, unsweetened (½ C)

VEGETABLES

(Raw, 1 C)

Cabbage

Celery

Chinese cabbage

Cucumber

Green onion

Hot peppers

Mushrooms

Radishes

Zucchini

SALAD GREENS

Endive

Escarole

Lettuce

Romaine

Spinach

SWEET SUBSTITUTES

Candy, hard, sugar-free

Gelatin, sugar-free

Gum, sugar-free

Jam/jelly, sugar-free (2 t)

Pancake syrup, sugar-free (1–2 T)

Sugar substitutes (saccharin, aspartame)

Whipped topping (2 T)

CONDIMENTS

Catsup (1 T)

Horseradish

Mustard

Pickles, dill, unsweetened

Salad dressing, low-calorie (2 T)

Taco sauce (1 T)

Vinegar

Seasonings can be very helpful in making food taste better. Be careful of how much sodium you use. Read the label, and choose those seasonings that do not contain sodium or salt.

Basil (fresh)	Garlic	Oregano
Cinnamon	Herbs	Pepper
Chili powder	Hot pepper sauce	Pimento
Chives	Lemon	Spices
Curry	Lemon juice	Soy sauce
Dill	Lemon pepper	Soy sauce, low-sodium
Flavoring extracts	Lime	("lite")
(vanilla, almond, walnut,	Lime juice	Wine, used in cooking
peppermint, lemon butter,	Mint	($1/4$ C)
etc.)	Onion powder	Worcestershire sauce

FOODS TO AVOID   Sugar, candy, honey, jam, jelly, marmalade, syrups, pie, cake, cookies, pastries, condensed milk, soft drinks, candy-coated gum; fried, scalloped or creamed foods; beer, wine or other alcoholic beverages.

---

nutritive sweeteners and calorie-free beverages have little or no carbohydrate, protein, or fat, and are therefore not restricted in any meal plan.

Here is an example of how to work the exchange lists. Let's say your doctor asks you to follow a 1,500-calorie diet that provides about 190 grams of carbohydrate, 60 grams of protein, and 40 grams of fat. You would turn to the nutrient summaries in each exchange list (item number 2 above). By mixing and matching various types of foods, you might come up with a daily list that looks like this:

7 starches
5 lean meats or meat alternatives
3 vegetables
3 fruits
2 skim milks
5 fats

The nutrient summary tells you that the foods on these exchange lists deliver 189 grams of carbohydrates, 57 grams of protein, 35 grams of fat, and 1,450 calories—just what the doctor ordered.

A sample menu to match this amount of food might look like this:

Morning	2 starches	1/2 cup grits and 1 slice toast
	1 fruit	1 fresh orange
	1 skim milk	8 oz skim milk
	1 fat	2 tsp reduced-fat (diet) margarine
	free foods	coffee or tea with sugar substitute
Midday	2 starches	2 slices bread
	2 meats	2 oz sliced turkey with mustard
	1 vegetable	1 cup vegetable soup
	free foods	large tossed salad
	1 fat	1 tbsp lowfat salad dressing
Snack	1 fruit	1 apple
Evening	2 starches	1/2 cup blackeyed peas and 1/3 cup brown rice
	3 meats	3 oz broiled fish
	2 vegetables	1/2 cup string beans
		1/2 cup stewed tomatoes
	1 fat	1 tsp reduced-fat margarine and 2 tsp reduced-fat salad dressing
	free foods	large salad and sliced cucumbers
		3/4 cup sugar-free gelatin dessert

Snack	1 starch	3 cups popcorn
	1 fat	cooked in 2 tsp oil
	1 skim milk	8 oz skim milk blended with
	1 fruit	1/2 ripe banana

To vary the menu for the next day, simply check the exchange lists and select different foods. The serving size of any food can be adjusted to fit an exchange.

If a food has a nutrition information label, note the following:

• what the portion size is;
• how many grams of carbohydrate, protein, and fat are in each portion;
• which exchange list it best fits.

Many new products labeled "sugar-free" may need special attention. Fortunately, many baked goods and other items that are sweetened with fruit juices describe each portion in terms of diabetic exchanges. Check the label. These may be welcome items in homes that have banned sugary junk foods.

However, use a different strategy if a bakery claims that a muffin, for example, is sugar-free. Ask them to explain how the item is sweetened. If it was baked with no sweetener or a nonnutritive sweetener, consider the muffin a starch or bread exchange. Every ounce is equivalent to a slice of bread (yes, it's helpful to weigh the muffin on a food scale). If the baker used a nutritive sweetener, you may want to consider the muffin a combination of one bread exchange and one half of a fruit exchange. If a well-meaning friend has baked a treat with a combination of sweeteners—say, part nonnutritive sweetener and part table sugar (sucrose), don't despair. As long as your serving contains less than one teaspoon of sugar, you're in the clear.

To use the exchange tables, you should have an idea of how many calories you want to eat in a day. Then consult Table 7, which will tell you how many exchanges of various foods you should eat to achieve your overall calorie goal.

WHEN YOU ARE SICK

When they are sick, especially when they have a fever, many diabetics find that their usual diets must be altered to satisfy their body's new needs. Fever or illness tend to raise blood glucose levels. That means you still need to take your insulin or your pills, even though you have cut back on your eating because your illness has taken your appetite. In fact, despite eating less food, most diabetics need *more* insulin during illnesses. The Joslin Clinic recommends this cardinal rule: *Never omit insulin or decrease the dose unless tests made every four hours show the urine to be free from acetone and free from glucose or nearly so.*

As you continue with your medication, keep monitoring your blood for glucose and your urine for ketones. If the levels change, notify your doctor. Your doctor should also advise you of medicines that are sugar-free or that do not elevate blood glucose levels.

Food and beverages are very important on sick days. It is important to eat the same amount of carbohydrate that you normally do, although on sick days you may want to spread your quota throughout

TABLE 7 Food Exchanges Recommended for Different Calorie Levels

	1300 calories 160 g carbohydrate (50%) 68 g protein (21%) 40 g fat (29%)	1500 calories 190 g carbohydrate (52%) 75 g protein (20%) 45 g fat (28%)	1800 calories 230 g carbohydrate (53%) 80 g protein (18%) 60 g fat (29%)	2100 calories carbohydrate(55%) 90 g protein (17%) 65 g fat (28%)
NUMBER OF EXCHANGES				
Starch	6	7	8	9
Meat (medium-fat)	4	5	5	6
Vegetables	3	3	3	3
Fruit	1	3	4	5
Skim milk	2	2	2	2
Fat	4	4	7	7

This chart, based on recent American Diabetes Association recommendations, should be taken to your own physician who will guide you to the best diet for your individual needs.

the day instead of having it in three meals. Try easy-to-manage foods such as crackers, toast, and mashed potato, in the portion sizes that correspond to the amount recommended in the exchange list.

Liquids are always an important part of everyone's diet, but they become especially crucial if you have a fever, vomiting, or diarrhea. If you are unable to eat, drink calorie-free liquids such as water, broth, or sugar-free soft drinks. Many people prefer to let the carbonation go flat before consuming soft drinks. Drink a minimum or four to eight ounces of these liquids every hour.

If you are having difficulty eating because of a sore throat or tender stomach, satisfy your normal carbohydrate quota with regular sodas, popsicles, juice, or soup. Try to spread out fifty grams of carbohydrates over three or four hours to prevent your blood sugar from dropping too low. If you can't tolerate even these foods, contact your doctor. It's a good idea to record everything you eat when you're sick. That way if you need to ask your doctor for help, you have a ready-made list of your entire recent diet.

Table 8 lists the carbohydrate content of foods in a sample "sick day" menu:

TABLE 8 "Sick Day" Foods

Amount to be eaten in 3 to 4 hours	Grams of carbohydrates
4 oz regular soda	10
1/2 twin bar popsicle	10
1/2 cup cooked cereal	15
6 saltine crackers	15
	50
6 oz apricot nectar	30
1 slice toast	15
1 cup broth	0
	45

The bread/starch exchanges and fruit exchanges will provide you with substantial carbohydrates. Oftentimes milk products are not well-tolerated if someone has a digestive tract upset such as diarrhea or vomiting.

MANAGING YOUR WEIGHT

By now, you already know that for the vast majority of African-Americans, weight control is the golden key to controlling diabetes. What's often less clear is how to lose the weight we don't want. The trick is to tip the energy equation in your favor by eating fewer calories than you burn up. That usually means making a significant change in your eating habits, so you need firm resolve to get started. Enlist the help of a registered dietician or other health care provider to set up a flexible, reasonable dietary plan. Avoid formulas, packaged diet plans, and weight-loss pills. The only thing they make lighter is your wallet. Once you have a sound dietary plan, ask a buddy or partner to help you overcome the emotional barriers. It's always easier to win a challenge when we have someone to cheer us on.

To lose weight reasonably and safely, try the following four-step plan.

Step #1: Calculate your ideal weight.

The amount that you should weigh may be much less than your current weight. Don't be discouraged. Be realistic. If you are one hundred pounds overweight, divide your overall goal into smaller pieces and set ten or twenty-five pounds as your first weight-loss goal. Achieving that will inspire you to move on to the next target. To find your recommended weight, turn to page 35.

Your doctor may suggest a particular weight-loss goal that is best for you.

Step #2: Calculate your daily calorie needs.

To find out approximately how many calories you need in a day, use Table 9. Note that you can use Table 9 to figure out how

TABLE 9 Recommended Calorie Needs per Pound of Body Weight

Body State/Goal	Sedentary	Active	Very Active
Overweight/weight loss	9–11	14	16
Normal weight/ weight maintenance	14	16	18
Underweight/weight gain	16	18	20–23

many calories you need to consume to lose weight. For example, let's say you weigh 200 pounds and you want to lose weight. You are sedentary. According to Table 9, you would need to eat about 10 calories per pound, or 10 x 200 = 2,000 calories each day.

Step #3: Use the exchange lists to plan menus that will satisfy your daily calorie goal.

Once you know that you need to consume no more than two thousand calories each day, for example, you can build a menu that holds the line at this number of calories while delivering all of the nutrients you need for good health. From Table 7 (page 100), you can see that two thousand calories falls closest to the twenty-one hundred-calorie breakdown in the right-most column. How could you get rid of those extra one hundred calories? You could eliminate one starch, which would save you eighty calories. Or you could cut out a medium meat exchange, for a savings of seventy-five calories. Either way would put you close to your goal of two thousand calories a day. Once you know how many of the various food exchanges you are allowed to eat, you can go about planning your daily menus.

Step #4: Be tough, but be patient.

The most difficult obstacle at the start of a weight-loss program is what dieticians call the "deprivation blues"—the longing we have for a larger piece of chicken, a second slice of pizza, another slice of sweet potato pie. The best defense against these cravings is to take the offensive. Treat yourself to special luxuries that have nothing to do with food: a hobby magazine, a movie, or even a hot relaxing bubble bath.

At the same time, "Push hard, especially at the beginning." That advice comes from Drs. Thomas Flood, medical director of the Atlanta Hospital and Regional Diabetes Center, and Ramachandiran Cooppan of the Joslin Clinic. "Most patients with Type 2 diabetes will both tolerate and benefit from a brief period of extremely restricted dieting at the onset of therapy." The doctors recommend an initial daily intake of six hundred to one thousand calories, plus vitamin and mineral supplements. After a short while, the diet is adjusted so that you lose one or two pounds per week. If your doctor or dietician agrees that this is a good approach for you, ask her or him how long you should stay in this initial low-calorie phase.

Why the two-phase approach? You might recall from Chapter 1 that the reason doctors advise weight loss for Type 2 diabetics has to do with changes inside your body's cells. When you're overweight, receptors on the surface of your cells don't respond very well to insulin. As you lose weight, the receptors regain their sensitivity, which lets your cells take in glucose like normal. The idea behind the initial sharp cutback in calories is to initiate this beneficial change in your receptor cells while at the same time not cause adverse effects.

The key to success is gradual weight loss—no more than one or two pounds each week. In fact, under the usual conditions of reduced calorie intake and increased activity, it's impossible to lose more than one or two pounds per week. The winners in the battle against excess weight are long-distance runners, not sprinters. Be patient.

The pounds that you lose add up. Each pound of body fat represents 3,500 calories. Thus if you eat 500 fewer calories each day, you will probably rid your body of one pound of fat each week. If you burn off 250 calories a day as exercise and omit 250 calories from your diet, you should reap a modest but steady loss each week. Remember, a pound a week amounts to 52 pounds over the course of a year.

Establishing a good, healthful diet is an excellent path to weight loss. But it's only half the picture. The other half—exercise—is absolutely essential for losing weight. You can eat well without exercising. And you can exercise without eating well. But in neither case will you lose weight, at least not permanently. It takes a two-pronged approach to get the results that you want.

For people with diabetes, exercise is extremely important for good health even if you're not trying to lose weight. Unfortunately, exercise is probably the most neglected tool in our arsenal against diabetes. You can probably guess why: many people simply don't enjoy exercising. But I have a hunch that more folks with diabetes would jump on the exercise bandwagon if they knew about the remarkable things it can do for them. And besides, I know a few tricks that will actually make exercise fun. Just turn the page.

EXERCISING
YOUR OPTIONS

The very mention of the word "exercise" strikes most patients—
and many physicians—with a sense of utter dread. We think of
our heart pounding so hard that it threatens to leap from our ribcage.
We picture being so out of breath that our entire being focuses on
gasping for air. We remember muscles whose soreness after a workout is rivaled only by their stiffness the next morning. As activities
go, I'm afraid exercise doesn't always have a sterling reputation.

Happily, exercise doesn't have to hurt. It doesn't need to be
painful. It doesn't have to feel like you're one step from certain
death. Indeed, I would argue that exercise should and can be fun.
But if you are one of the many who have difficulty imagining "fun"
and "exercise" in the same sentence, I ask that you imagine the following scenario.

Let's say you're picking up some insulin at your pharmacy, and
the pharmacist asks if you've heard of a brand new medicine for
diabetes. The new drug lowers blood sugar levels dramatically—
tenfold or more. And that's just the beginning. This new wonder
drug helps guard against no less than seven additional health problems that typically plague African-American diabetics—atherosclerosis, heart attacks, obesity, blood disorders, hypertension, insulin
resistance, and stress. Best of all, the medicine is so user-friendly
that taking the drug is actually enjoyable.

With today's high price of prescription drugs, you might expect to pay a handsome sum for medicine whose reach and effectiveness are so vast. But this medicine comes free of charge: it's exercise.

Exercise, the second leg of our three-legged stool, brings wondrous benefits to people with diabetes. Exercise has been used to help people with diabetes for at least twenty-five hundred years. According to one early medical text, physicians in India were prescribing exercise for diabetics as early as 500 B.C. In the first century A.D., a Roman scientist named Celsus also advocated exercise for diabetes. In the years that followed, exercise fluctuated in popularity. As recently as a century ago, many physicians thought people with diabetes were too fragile to exercise.

But in the past seventy years, with the resurgence of interest in diabetes treatment that followed the discovery of insulin, doctors began looking at exercise with renewed hope. And since the 1970s, when studies finally nailed down the risks and benefits of exercise in diabetes, physicians have placed increasing faith in exercise and recommended it to untold thousands of patients.

Clearly, exercise doesn't have precisely the same effects in all diabetics, any more than it works the same magic in all persons without diabetes. And no one has yet studied the specific effects of exercise in African-Americans. But black Americans should take note of a transformation underway in the Zuni tribe in Arizona, where diabetes is widespread. Researchers have been working with the Zuni to incorporate running and other forms of exercise into their daily lives. The hope is that regular physical activity can help to both prevent and treat diabetes. The new routine seems to be working. The Zuni have a popular saying these days: "Ho Chikwa: Weykkya Hanukwa." Translation: "I outran diabetes."

THE BENEFITS OF EXERCISE

If you are prone to diabetes—if the disease runs in your family, for example—but you don't have the disease, exercise can reduce your chances of becoming a diabetic. Regular exercise reduces the risk of getting diabetes by an estimated 41 percent in middle-aged men, according to research at the University of Pennsylvania. These findings are believed equally valid for women. Every five hundred calories that the men burned each week while exercising decreased their diabetes risk another 6 percent.

If you already have diabetes, exercise helps your body handle glucose by removing the sugar from the bloodstream and making your tissues more sensitive to insulin. And it guards against the many complications of atherosclerosis (thickening and hardening of the arteries). These two benefits alone help guarantee diabetics longer, healthier lives. In addition, exercise can also help you lose weight, and it is wonderfully calming—a surefire help for those of us who get stressed out (and who doesn't?). Before we discuss how to go about starting an exercise regimen, let's take a closer look at what exercise does for diabetics and how this desirable transformation takes place.

Better Glucose Management

You are sitting on an exercise bicycle, breathing hard but feeling good. For the past twenty minutes, you've pedaled a steady rhythm, enough to work up a light sweat. As you head for the shower, you feel relaxed and proud. And if you could look inside your bloodstream, you'd be even more gratified. Much of the glucose that was in your blood when you started pedaling—glucose that was present in worrisome high amounts—has suddenly left your bloodstream.

This is a hypothetical scenario, but it's based in fact. Exercise shakes up the body's mechanism for using glucose. In people without diabetes, exercise increases the amount of glucose demanded by the muscles and other tissues by a factor of ten or more. When we start to exercise, the pancreas senses the need for more glucose and releases less insulin. The decline in insulin production prompts the liver to release glucose into the bloodstream. From the bloodstream, these backup supplies of sugar flow directly into the tissues that need them.

This same mechanism works for people with diabetes. Exercise seems to reverse the resistance that makes a person's tissues unresponsive to insulin. Do you remember in Chapter 1 how I compared insulin resistance to a mail carrier arriving at your home but finding the mailbox welded shut? Exercise releases those welds, thus allowing insulin to bring glucose into the tissues again. In fact, when people with mild diabetes follow a strenuous program of exercising five or more times a week for a year, their glucose tolerance often becomes completely normal. This is the type of discovery that convinces doctors that we will soon be able to prevent diabetes.

Diabetics don't have to work this hard to reap the glucose-regulating effects of exercise. Moderately strenuous exercise several times a week can work wonders to reverse insulin resistance, especially when combined with weight loss. This beneficial effect lasts for some time after you stop exercising. For as many as twelve hours after an exercise session, your body continues to smoothly shuttle glucose into your tissues. So the benefits of a single workout can carry over through the next several meals.

If you take insulin, chances are you won't need as much of it if you exercise. Exercise does such a good job of clearing a path for bloodstream glucose to enter your tissues that diabetics often discover their need for insulin declines. When diabetic children go to summer camp, they often return home using less insulin than they did when they left because of the heightened physical activity there. Doctors know that a patient who is hospitalized needs less insulin after their discharge because people get more exercise at home.

Exercise is good for you, even if you happen to be hospitalized. Bed rest is hard on the body. Once you stop exercising your muscles, they begin to deteriorate immediately, although most people don't notice it for several weeks. You begin to slowly lose bone, which can contribute to osteoporosis, or "brittle bones." And of course, your body becomes less efficient at handling glucose. Since a hospital stay can be prolonged—the average stay for a diabetic hospitalized with a foot ulcer in 1985 was six weeks—exercising is a must.

Lower Risk of Atherosclerosis

When you have lots of glucose in your bloodstream, you'll recall, the sugar adheres to blood proteins and forms sticky clumps that can clog your blood vessels. Conversely, anything that lowers the amount of glucose in your blood might reduce your risk of developing atherosclerosis by this route. Exercise, by its ability to send glucose away from the bloodstream and into your tissues, is one way of getting this assistance.

As a matter of fact, exercise helps prevent thickened, hardened arteries in a number of ways. For example, exercise lowers the bloodstream levels of a substance known as VLDL—very low density lipoprotein, a form of cholesterol. Scientists don't know if VLDL contributes to atherosclerosis (like its cousin LDL does). But they do know that in people with diabetes, VLDL can change to a form that makes it more likely to cause this cardiovascular disease. Because exercise reduces the amount of VLDL in your blood, it also reduces your risk of atherosclerosis.

Exercise seems to help normalize blood clotting. Diabetes causes blood to clot more than it should, because it makes certain clot-producing blood cells overactive. This can lead to the formation of fatty plaque seen in thickened, clogged arteries. Doctors find that Type 2 diabetics who begin a program of regular exercise enjoy more normal blood clotting in as little as six weeks.

Lower Blood Pressure

High blood pressure, a special problem in diabetics and a condition that worsens atherosclerosis, improves with exercise. As a rule, people who are more active have lower blood pressure than those who are sedentary. After four months of regular exercise, Type 2 diabetics who were eating well enjoyed a drop in average diastolic blood pressure of ten to fifteen points in tests by researchers from the University of Medicine and Dentistry of New Jersey/Robert Wood Johnson Medical School and the Boston University School of Medicine.

Less Stress

African-American diabetics, like most African-Americans, live stressful lives. Stress can elevate your blood glucose and is thought to heighten the risk of atherosclerosis. Exercise, as you probably know, is one of the best stress-relievers we have. Studies show that exercise helps moderate our body's responses to stresses, while helping to lift depression. "Most studies suggest that regular exercise results in improved mood, decreased anxiety, and a more positive self-image," suggests Dr. Neil Ruderman of the Boston University Medical School, who has studied the benefits of exercise for African-Americans who have Type 2 diabetes. These benefits, in turn, might help people stick with their daily routine of watching their diet, taking their medicine, and monitoring their blood sugar.

Weight Loss

Perhaps the most important benefit of regular exercise, at least for black folks, is weight loss. Excess body weight is associated not only with atherosclerosis but with a host of other disorders ranging from heart disease and arthritis to diabetes, of course, and even cancer. If you combine reasonable calorie restrictions (as spelled out in Chapter 6) with regular, moderate exercise, the resulting weight loss can benefit your health tremendously. Just as obesity increases insulin resistance, making it difficult for glucose to find its way into your cells, weight loss normalizes insulin resistance, thus restoring the healthy metabolism of glucose and reducing a buildup of sugar in your bloodstream. This is why weight loss is the very first strategy that doctors recommend to their overweight Type 2 diabetics.

While many aspects of diabetes are not fully understood, the evidence for the benefits of weight loss is crystal clear. If because of your genetic makeup you are resistant to insulin, you are five to ten times more likely to develop diabetes, according to one estimate. At the Joslin Clinic, which tracks diabetes in various populations, about half of the people in one study were resistant to insulin but didn't have diabetes. Dr. Ronald Kahn and colleagues found that over the years, every person who eventually developed diabetes was insulin-resistant. "The factor that most clearly predicts who will develop diabetes is insulin resistance," Dr. Kahn told the *New York Times.*

But Dr. Kahn also discovered that the people who were insulin-resistant and hadn't become overweight lowered their risk of developing diabetes. Even after a person had grown overweight, losing weight reduced their risk of developing diabetes to the point that they were only slightly more likely to get the disease than were members of the general population. This means that we can greatly lessen our odds of getting diabetes—even if we are genetically prone to diabetes—by slimming down if we're overweight, or by not becoming overweight in the first place.

Exercise can play an important role in both. Exercise encourages your body to burn calories faster by revving up your internal furnace. Some studies show that this boost in your metabolism rate does more than simply burn up calories while you are exercising. Indeed, the higher metabolic rate persists for hours after you stop exercising. That means each exercise workout keeps your internal thermostat humming along, burning calories left and right. And as we all know, the key to losing weight is burning more calories than we take in.

All things considered, regular exercise may add years to your life. After all, atherosclerosis and its many complications (heart disease, kidney failure, nerve damage, stroke, and so forth) are responsible for much of why Type 2 diabetics die before their time.

When doctors say that the person who determines the course of diabetes is the patient, not the doctor, this is what they mean. Only you can decide to eat a beneficial diet, and only you can stick with a program of regular exercise. The benefits of doing so are overwhelming, and I hope you'll take the plunge with enthusiasm.

BEFORE YOU EXERCISE

If you have diabetes, no matter how old you are, you must check with your doctor before you start any exercise program. If you are over thirty years of age, or you have had diabetes for more than ten years, your doctor may want to give you a thorough cardiovascular evaluation. This may include a stress test, during which you will be asked to walk a treadmill while monitors measure how well your heart responds to the exercise. A stress test can be a lifesaver; it typically reveals heart disease in 10 percent of the diabetics who otherwise have no symptoms. If you are suffering any complications from diabetes, your doctor will want to decide whether it's safe for you to go ahead, or whether it's better to wait until the complications clear up. Once you have been evaluated, your doctor will suggest how long your workouts should last, how hard you should push yourself, and how often you should exercise.

CHOOSING AN EXERCISE

The choice of exercise is usually left to you. There are two basic kinds of exercise: aerobic and anaerobic. Aerobic exercise stimulates the heart and lungs by involving large numbers of muscles. Walking and running are good aerobic exercises, as are swimming and bicycling. Here's a more complete list:

AEROBIC EXERCISES

INDIVIDUAL ACTIVITIES	TEAM SPORTS	
Brisk walking	Badminton	Soccer
Running/jogging	Golf	Basketball
Bicycling (incl. stationary)	Wrestling	Volleyball
Swimming	Fencing	Hockey
Dancing	Stair climbing	(field and ice)
Rope skipping	Calisthenics	Lacrosse
Skiing (downhill and cross-country)	Tennis	
	Handball	
Rowing	Squash	
Skating	Racquetball	

SOURCE: Marble A., et al., *Joslin's Diabetes Mellitus*, 12th ed., Philadelphia: Lea & Febiger, 1985, p. 457. Used with permission.

Walking is a particularly valuable sport, especially for older or more sedentary diabetics. Brisk walking is a good heart conditioner that requires little or no equipment, and carries little risk of overtaxing the heart. Of course, remember to continue to treat your feet with kid gloves. If your feet have open sores, wait until they are healed before you take up walking. And if you have a corn, a callus, a bunion, or an ingrown toenail, see your doctor or a podiatrist before you hit the trail. He or she may recommend special shoes to help protect your feet.

For years, doctors have recommended aerobic exercise for people with diabetes, because this is the type of exercise that improves insulin sensitivity and reduces the amount of glucose in the blood. Recent evidence suggests that anaerobic exercise—exercise like weight-lifting that increases muscle strength but doesn't give your heart and lungs a good workout—may also help the body handle glucose. But people injure themselves more often doing anaerobic exercise, and they may not enjoy all of the benefits of aerobic workouts. So for the best of the benefits without so many risks, aerobic exercise is the better way to go.

Pick an exercise that you enjoy, one that you can envision doing several times a week without getting bored. Or pick more than one exercise and alternate. As long as your workouts satisfy some basic criteria (explained below), it doesn't matter how you work up a sweat.

One special note: if you live in the inner city, exercise can pose a special challenge. I remember one of my patients, a fifty-year-old diabetic, who took up jogging in his urban neighborhood. Two weeks later, he showed up in our clinic on crutches, having been assaulted on one of his outings. We arranged for him to exercise in our hospital gymnasium, and control of his diabetes became excellent.

Jogging or running in the streets can be dangerous in some neighborhoods. Admission to hospital exercise facilities is limited, and exercise equipment may be more expensive than inner-city residents can afford. It may take ingenuity by both patient and doctor to build an exercise program that's safe and affordable. One option if you live in an apartment building or a home: stair climbing. It's an excellent aerobic exercise.

How Long to Exercise

Plan to spend at least fifteen to twenty minutes of solid exercise each time you have a session. Anything less than fifteen or twenty minutes doesn't do much good; more than forty-five minutes of exercising increases the chance of injury. But don't just put in your twenty minutes and rush off. For best results and to minimize the chance of injuring your muscles, take time before and after the session to warm up and cool down. Dr. Hassan Kanj of the University of Medicine and Dentistry of New Jersey/Robert Wood Johnson Medical School recommends ten minutes of stretching initially, followed by five to ten minutes of easy warm-up exercise. The warm-up can be a slower, gentler version of the same exercise that you do more strenuously later in the session. Then comes the heart of your workout—fifteen to twenty minutes of work. Afterwards, five or ten minutes of warm-down exercise.

How Hard to Exercise

The cardiovascular benefits of exercise begin only after your heartbeat climbs above a certain rate. The rate you should aim for depends on several factors. If you are young and active, and if you haven't had diabetes for very long, your doctor may allow you to exercise all-out. This may mean working out hard enough to bring your heart rate within 80 to 90 percent of its maximum rate. If you are older or sedentary, if you aren't controlling diabetes as well as you could, or if you have certain complications, your doctor will want you to start slowly. You may be advised to aim for 60 to 70 percent of your maximum heart rate.

Your maximum heart rate depends on your age. Use the heart rate chart (Table 10) to find the heart rate you should try to achieve during exercise. For example, if you are a Type 2 diabetic who is forty-five years old, and you are relatively out of shape, you should aim for 60 to 70 percent of your maximum heart rate, or 108 to 126 beats per minute. To measure your heart rate during exercise, touch your finger to the pulse on either side of your throat. Count the beats for ten seconds, then multiply by six to get the rate per minute.

TABLE 10 Heart Rate During Exercise

Age	Maximum Heart Rate	60% of Maximum Rate	70% of Maximum Rate	80% of Maximum Rate	90% of Maximum Rate
15	193	116	135	154	174
20	191	115	134	153	172
25	189	113	133	151	170
30	186	111	130	149	167
35	184	110	129	147	166
40	182	109	127	146	164
45	180	108	126	144	162
50	178	107	125	142	160
55	175	105	123	140	158
60	173	104	121	138	156
65	171	103	120	137	154

SOURCE: Marble A., et al., *Joslin's Diabetes Mellitus*, 12th ed., Philadelphia: Lea & Febiger, 1985, p. 459. Used with permission.

Try to be aware of how your body feels as you work through these exercise sessions. If you try, you can develop a keen sensitivity to how your body responds to exercise at various levels of intensity. In time, you will know when to push yourself and when to let up. If you feel dull aches or fatigue, these are probably normal signs of newly worked muscles being put through their paces. If you feel sharp pain, that's your signal to slow down or stop; you may be on the verge of an injury. When your body feels "comfortable" at a certain level, you may increase the intensity of your workout to raise your heart rate. In time, and with your doctor's permission, you can progress from the 60 percent rate to the 80 to 90 percent rate.

How Often to Exercise

Exercise three to five times a week to obtain the benefits of better blood-sugar control. Exercise more—anywhere from five to seven times a week—if you want to lose weight. You might be tempted to compensate for fewer exercise sessions by exercising more intensely. It doesn't work. Whether to bring about better blood-sugar control or to lose weight, your body needs the benefits that only steady repetition can bring.

When to Exercise

Exercise whenever it's comfortable for you. Early morning sessions before breakfast are particularly beneficial. That way, the twelve hours of enhanced glucose management can benefit you throughout the day. If you do choose to exercise during the day, wait at least an hour after eating. That will give your body a chance to reduce the high blood sugar levels that follow a meal. Exercising in the evening carries the risk of developing hypoglycemia (low blood sugar) overnight.

Before Each Exercise Session

Check your blood sugar and monitor your urine before you begin each exercise session. If your blood sugar is higher than 240 milligrams per deciliter, or if you find ketones in your urine, wait until your blood sugar falls and you are eliminating no ketones.

Cautions About Exercise

If you are a diabetic, starting an exercise program doesn't change the fact that you have diabetes. Unlike nondiabetics, you must approach exercise fully aware of several possible complications that can stem from the impact of exercise on your body.

HYPOGLYCEMIA   The most common complication is low blood sugar. Exercise normally doesn't reduce the levels of blood glucose for a nondiabetic, because the liver contributes glucose from stockpiles of glycogen. But in diabetics, strenuous exercise on an empty stomach can cause blood sugar to plummet, sometimes for hours afterwards. Sometimes this sharp drop in blood sugar is a delayed reaction that doesn't happen until eighteen to twenty-four hours after the exercise session.

To help guard against hypoglycemia, eat a snack containing ten or fifteen grams (one-half ounce) of a simple carbohydrate thirty minutes before you exercise. If your exercise session will be particularly intense, add five grams. Use snacks only if your blood glucose level is under 150 milligrams per deciliter. During the exercise session, you can eat an additional fifteen to thirty grams of carbohydrate every half hour. After exercising, a final snack of a slowly absorbed carbohydrate (such as milk or a starch) can help you avoid delayed hypoglycemia.

Another way to guard against hypoglycemia is to remember that exercise reduces your need for insulin. If you use insulin, reduce your dose before you exercise, particularly if your workout will be unusually taxing.

EYE PROBLEMS   If you have diabetic retinopathy, avoid vigorous or intense exercise, or jarring exercises (jumping rope, running, dancing), which can sometimes worsen this condition. Also avoid weight-lifting and other exercises that raise blood pressure in your head. Before you start exercising, ask an ophthalmologist for advice. He or she may want to treat the condition with laser therapy before allowing you to begin.

FOOT INJURY   If you have nerve damage, you may inadvertently injure your feet. Avoid exercises (like jogging) that subject your feet to repeated pounding. Wear comfortable, padded footwear and inspect your feet carefully after exercising.

OVERCOMING OBSTACLES

The many rewards of exercise—gaining greater physical endurance, increasing your emotional well-being, losing weight, delaying or avoiding complications of diabetes—are so sizable that many diabetics start exercising programs with enthusiasm and incorporate them into their daily lives for years. Others find it more difficult to start exercising, or have difficulty maintaining their good health habits once they have begun. It's only natural and human that you find yourself confronted with one obstacle or another as you try to launch an exercise effort or keep one going. Here's some advice on how you can leap those hurdles and keep up your good work.

FIND AN EXERCISE PARTNER   As anyone who has tried to lose weight will tell you, the pounds are much easier to put on than they are to take off. Being black makes weight loss even more challenging. Why? For one thing, black folks have historically viewed fatness as a positive sign. Food supplies aren't always predictable in Africa, so our ancestors learned to equate plumpness with prosperity. In addition, older black men and women are more likely to face disabilities that make exercising difficult. In one study at the University of South Carolina, elderly blacks had twice as much difficulty as elderly whites did with such everyday tasks as dressing, eating, and walking unassisted across a room. To a person who finds it hard to even dress, the prospect of calisthenics or a brisk walk around the block might sound like fantasy.

And yet African-Americans of all ages and a variety of stages of disability can and do enjoy the benefits of regular exercise. In fact, many with disabilities find that exercise diminishes their pain and restores motion to their joints. For people with disabilities, a good occupational therapist can help people restore much of the body's lost strength and flexibility. For all of us, one good way to overcome societal pressures against exercise is to find a partner to exercise with. A partner can be a neighbor, a friend, a sibling, someone who's fat or thin. The important thing is that they share your commitment to exercise.

Once you have an exercise partner, you can do as much or as little with them as you want. You can walk to the gym or the park and exercise together. You can compare notes and keep track of each other's progress. If you haven't exercised in years, you can even commiserate about your creaky bones. Somehow, having a buddy go through the experience with you makes exercise immensely more pleasurable. It also keeps you motivated to continue when your willpower might otherwise wilt.

STAY ACTIVE   Some dieters feel entitled to a big dish of pie á la mode just because they washed down their lunch with a low-calorie soda. That's counterproductive, because the dessert contains many more calories than you could ever save by drinking a diet beverage. Likewise, don't assume that exercising means you can continue an otherwise sedentary lifestyle as long as you stroll a few laps around the track each morning. For exercise to be a part of a successful weight-loss program, you must make exercise just one part of an overall effort to be more active.

Dr. F. Xavier Pi-Sunyer, president of the American Diabetes Association and an obesity researcher, discovered that when overweight people join exercise programs, they tend to be less active once they finish each day's workout. Since people who are sedentary burn fewer calories than people who are active, this inactivity negates much of the weight lost through an exercise program. If you exercise, do it as part of a larger effort toward a more active lifestyle.

ABOVE ALL, HAVE FUN   This advice may sound strange after reading cautions about diabetics and exercise. But if you can manage to relax and inject an element of play in your workout, you will think of exercise as more fun than work. "Study after study shows that the people who stick with exercise are the ones who really enjoy their activity," writes Carol Krucoff in the *Washington Post*. "They don't view their workout as one more chore to cram in but as a play break that's one of the highlights of their day."

Exercise as play isn't a new idea. When we were children, all of our exercise was fun. Running, hopping, biking, skating—life was a huge playground, and exercise came so naturally that we never thought of it as work.

How can we recapture the fun in exercise? One way is to think back to what was fun for us as children. Did you enjoy hikes through the woods? Maybe you'd enjoy a quiet walk through your neighborhood at dawn (if it's safe), or a brisk jaunt through a nearby meadow or park. Did you ever fantasize about being the next Arnold Palmer? Maybe returning to the fairways would bring back pleasant memories. Were you a lifeguard at summer camp? Maybe some laps at the Y are just what you need to refresh your spirit.

Have fun.

TAKING YOUR MEDICINE

One evening a patient of mine summoned me to the home of a sick neighbor. When I arrived, the woman was weak, in a stupor, and breathing slowly and deeply. Urine in a chamber pot tested strongly positive for glucose and ketones. We rushed her to a hospital where she was found to be in a diabetic coma. When we gave the patient insulin and appropriate fluids, she responded beautifully. Without insulin, she would have died.

Such is the legacy of modern medicine, the great strides we have made to help the body cope with diabetes.

By odd coincidence, the world's most important diabetes breakthroughs have coincided with global conflict. The first useful extracts of insulin for humans were prepared in 1921, a few years after World War I. A second major breakthrough—the development of pancreas-boosting pills called *sulfonylureas* (sul´fo-nil-yu-re´-az)—came in 1945 at the conclusion of World War II. Despite the backdrop of war, these discoveries brought diabetics throughout the world enormous peace. After generations of impotence against diabetes, doctors finally had medicines that could often slow and sometimes even halt the progression of a dreaded killer.

Today, medication forms an important safety net for diabetics. The best way to control Type 2 diabetes is by modifying your lifestyle—losing weight, eating wisely, exercising regularly. When a patient can't achieve these goals, doctors prescribe medication. Diabetes pills are the first line of defense. These often reduce bloodstream sugar to manageable levels. If pills fail, insulin injections form a second strand of the safety net.

Over one million Americans take insulin at least once a day; nearly two million take diabetes pills, and around three million manage their diabetes solely by eating well. These represent about half of the twelve million diabetics in the United States; the others receive no treatment.

IF YOUR DOCTOR PRESCRIBES DIABETES PILLS

Most Americans think of medicine as something in bottles. Yet for hundreds of years, people in the rest of the world have found their medicines in plants. So when the earliest healers realized that diabetes is a disease of high blood sugar and set off in search of a remedy, they turned to the natural world that had already provided scores of effective remedies for human ailments. In the nonindustrialized world, these traditional remedies for diabetes remain popular today. The variety is extraordinary: from blueberry leaf extract to a fungus that grows on avocado plants. "Scarcely any physician interested in diabetes worldwide has not had a patient bring him from some unknown source a packet of dried leaves that were said to lower blood glucose," wrote Dr. Leo P. Krall as president of the International Diabetes Federation. And many of these natural remedies actually do reduce blood sugar, according to studies.

In its own way, the western arsenal against high blood sugar shows a bit of that same flash. Of the several dozen oral diabetes drugs worldwide, the six available in the United States are brightly colored torquoise tablets, pastel ovals, white diamonds, pink disks (Table 11). Like a lemon stimulates the flow of saliva in your mouth, these medicines act on the pancreas to stimulate the flow of insulin. Once insulin carries glucose from the bloodstream, the medicines conveniently find the door to the cells and open it, allowing glucose to enter.

WHO TAKES DIABETES PILLS   The typical patient who takes pills for diabetes develops the disease after reaching the age of forty, and has had diabetes for fewer than ten years. This is because the pills often lose effectiveness over time, either because the body isn't as responsive as it used to be or the diabetes worsens. Sometimes doctors prescribe these medicines in tandem with insulin. Most of these patients who use both insulin and pills take no more than twenty to thirty units of insulin.

The younger you are, the greater the chances that your doctor will prescribe insulin instead of pills. A National Health Interview Survey found that young adults with diabetes used insulin over pills by a margin of two to one (30 percent used insulin and 15 percent used pills). By middle age (age forty to fifty-nine), more patients were using pills (36 percent versus 21 percent on insulin). And by the time patients reached age sixty, they used pills over insulin by a margin of three to one (50 percent used pills and 17 percent used insulin).

TABLE 11 Pills That Lower Blood Sugar

Medicine	How it is sold	Usual starting dose*	Usual daily dose*
Diabeta	1.25 mg 2.5 mg 5 mg	2.5–5 mg	1.25–20 mg
Diabinese	100 mg 250 mg	250 mg	100–500 mg
Glucotrol	5 mg 10 mg	5 mg	less than 40 mg
Micronase	1.25 mg 2.5 mg 5 mg	2.5–5 mg	1.25–20 mg
Tolinase	100 mg 250 mg 500 mg	100–250 mg	100–1,000 mg

*Milligrams per day

WHO SHOULDN'T TAKE DIABETES PILLS   There are times when diabetes pills shouldn't be prescribed. If you have Type 1 diabetes, you shouldn't be taking sulfonylurea medicines. Diabeta, Glucotrol, and the four other pills in this family of medicines are only good for Type 2 diabetes.

If you have liver or kidney disease, your body may not be able to break down the pills and flush them from your system. Diabetes medicine can hurt unborn children, and it also winds up in a mother's breast milk. So these pills are not a good idea for pregnant or breastfeeding women, who are sometimes switched over to insulin during pregnancy, delivery, and breastfeeding. Finally, diabetes pills are not advised for diabetics in times of infection, surgery, illness, or other major stresses.

SIDE EFFECTS   Diabetes pills cause few side effects. A few patients notice upset stomachs, fever, or lack of energy, but side effects are rare.

THINGS TO BE CAREFUL ABOUT   Under certain conditions, diabetes pills can cause dangerous hypoglycemia, or low blood sugar. This can happen if you're elderly or malnourished, if you've recently consumed alcohol, if you have undergone a period of severe or prolonged exercise, or if you've either taken more than one glucose-lowering drug or too much of one drug.

Diabetes medicine can interact with other medicines to cause side effects. One example is a large class of drugs called *nonsteroidal anti-inflammatory medicines*. The most popular nonsteroidal anti-inflammatory drug is ibuprofen, which is found in Advil, Motrin, and Nuprin, and other popular medicines prescribed for pain and rheumatoid arthritis. These anti-inflammatory medicines can accentuate the effects of diabetes pills, so if you use ibuprofen while you take diabetes pills, keep a watchful eye for signs of low blood sugar.

Other medicines that tend to cause high blood sugar should be watched, too, because they can complicate your job of keeping your blood sugar low enough to be safe. Among the many glucose-raising drugs on the market are certain diuretics (urine-producers), thyroid medicines, oral contraceptives, estrogen, and calcium-channel blockers (for high blood pressure). If you are having trouble keeping your blood sugar low enough despite taking diabetes pills, and particularly if you recently switched to a new medicine, ask your doctor if the new medicine may be hurting your efforts to control your blood sugar.

Likewise, be careful if you stop taking a glucose-raising medicine while you are taking diabetes pills. You may be so accustomed to compensating for the extra blood sugar that once the glucose-raising medication is taken away, the pills make your blood sugar plummet.

IF YOUR DOCTOR PRESCRIBES INSULIN

Since its discovery in 1921, insulin has been given to millions of diabetics. This is not a rare drug that doctors and patients encounter only occasionally. Yet insulin is often prescribed and used improperly. "All too often insulin is not employed when needed or if taken, it is not used in a way and in such a dosage as to yield optimal results," says Dr. Alexander Marble, clinical professor emeritus of medicine at Harvard Medical School. "It is not uncommon for patients to be treated with diet alone or with oral hypoglycemic agents despite consistently poor results in the control of diabetes. Conversely, many patients are treated with insulin in the presence of obesity when the better policy would be to encourage loss of body weight by careful following of a hypocaloric [low-calorie] diet."

WHO SHOULD USE INSULIN   When is insulin a good idea? If you have Type 1 diabetes, insulin is for you. It doesn't matter when your diabetes began; insulin is appropriate for persons who developed Type 1 diabetes at any age—as children, teens, young adults, and occasionally even over age forty.

If you have Type 2 diabetes that simply cannot be controlled any other way, either by diet and exercise, or by diabetes pills, insulin is the way to go. Even if you are successfully controlling Type 2 diabetes, a doctor may still prescribe insulin when your body is facing the stresses of surgery or illness.

If you are pregnant and you have diabetes, you should take insulin. About 3 to 5 percent of women develop diabetes midway through their pregnancies. Their pancreas produces insulin just fine, but important hormones made by the placenta prevents insulin from working properly. We'll discuss diabetes during pregnancy in the next chapter.

WHAT KINDS OF INSULIN ARE AVAILABLE There are dozens of insulin preparations on the market. One of the most important differences among them is how quickly they act. *Regular* and *Semilente* (semi-len´tay) are fast-acting insulins. Once you inject them, they start working in as few as thirty minutes and they usually reach their peak activity an hour or two later. Because Regular is the fastest-working insulin, it is used in diabetic emergencies. *NPH* and *Lente* (len´tay) are intermediate-acting insulins. They start working an hour or two after you inject them, and reach their peak activity somewhere around three to ten hours later. *Ultralente* (ultra-len´tay) is the longest-acting insulin. It is slow to start working, but it stays active for over twenty-four hours.

Regular insulin was the only form available to diabetics for years after insulin was discovered; it is still the most popular insulin today. Because different insulin preparations have different amounts of "staying power," your doctor may direct you to use a mixture of two insulins, which can give you the coverage of both. Some insulin preparations come premixed; otherwise your doctor will show you how to mix your own.

HOW TO DETERMINE THE STRENGTH OF INSULIN Insulin comes in several strengths: U-40, U-100, and U-500. These designate the number of units of insulin contained in one milliliter of the hormone. Most insulin sold in the United States is U-100.

WHERE INSULIN COMES FROM Commercial insulin comes from any of several sources. Insulin has been traditionally extracted from the pancreas of cows or pigs. Biochemically speaking, these animals are similar enough to humans that their insulin performs in the human bloodstream just as our own insulin does.

Animal insulin typically contains tiny amounts of a protein called proinsulin. Insulin can legally contain up to .001 percent proinsulin; those products that do are labeled "Standard" insulin. Products that have been refined to reduce the proinsulin level to less than .0001 percent are labeled "Purified."

Starting in 1983 human insulin joined pork and beef insulin on the market. If you're wondering if human insulin is somehow squeezed from people's pancreas glands, let me reassure you—the answer is no. Human insulin is produced in one of two ways. Either pork insulin (which is nearly identical in structure to human insulin) is chemically altered to produce an identical twin of human insulin. Or harmless bacteria are programmed to produce human insulin through a process known as genetic engineering.

There is no evidence that human insulin works any better than animal insulin. All insulin, regardless of the source, is equally effective at lowering blood sugar levels. But by the same token, *insulin preparations are not interchangeable.* So don't switch from your prescribed insulin to another formula unless your doctor says so.

When your pharmacist hands you a bottle of insulin, double-check to make sure it is what your doctor specified. Look at the label. It will have the brand name (such as Humulin) and a large letter showing how fast-acting the product is. R stands for Regular, N stands for NPH, L stands for Lente, S stands for Semilente, and U stands for Ultralente. The label will tell you how strong the insulin is by clearly showing U-40 or U-100. Check the bottletop, too: U-40 bottles have red tops; U-100 bottles have orange tops.

Table 12 compares the nine types of animal and human insulin according to their effects on the body.

Table 13 shows insulin products available in the United States, along with the manufacturer, the form, and the strength of each product.

HOW TO ADMINISTER INSULIN Your doctor will explain how to measure the proper dose of insulin. The dose will be based on a combination of factors, including your current blood glucose reading and any anticipated demands on your body, such as forthcoming meals or exercise. Just as it's important to give yourself

TABLE 12 Action of Insulins

Type of Insulin	How quickly it starts to work (hours)	When peak action occurs (hours)	How long it is effective (hours)	How long it stays in your body (hours)
Human				
Regular	1/2–1	2–3	3–6	4–6
NPH	2–4	4–10	10–16	14–18
Lente	3–4	4–12	12–18	16–20
Ultralente	6–10	unknown	18–20	20–30
Animal				
Regular	1/2–2	3–4	4–6	6–8
Semilente	1–2	3–8	10–16	10–16
NPH	4–6	8–14	16–20	20–24
Lente	4–6	8–14	16–20	20–24
Ultralente	8–14	minimal	24–36	24–36

SOURCE: Reprinted with permission from *Diabetes Forecast*, October 1992, p. 39. Copyright © 1992 by American Diabetes Association, Inc.

TABLE 13 Insulin Available in the United States

Product	Company that makes it	Type of insulin	Where it comes from	How strong it is
Rapid-acting human insulin				
Humulin R	Lilly	Regular	bacteria	U-100
Humulin BR	Lilly	Regular	bacteria	U-100
Novolin R	Novo Nordisk	Regular	bacteria	U-100
Novolin R Penfill	Novo Nordisk	Regular	bacteria	U-100
Velosulin Human	Novo Nordisk	Regular	bacteria	U-100
Animal insulin				
Iletin II	Lilly	Regular	beef	U-100
Iletin II	Lilly	Regular	pork	U-100, U-500
Purified Pork R	Novo Nordisk	Regular	pork	U-100
Velosulin	Novo Nordisk	Regular	pork	U-100
Iletin I	Lilly	Regular	beef/pork	U-100
Regular	Novo Nordisk	Regular	pork	U-100
Iletin I Semilente	Lilly	Semilente	beef/pork	U-100
Semilente	Novo Nordisk	Semilente	beef	U-100
Rapid/intermediate-acting mixture				
Human insulin				
Humulin 70/30	Lilly	70% NPH, 30% Regular	bacteria	U-100
Humulin 50/50	Lilly	50% NPH, 50% Regular	bacteria	U-100

Continued on page 128

Mixtard Human 70/30	Novo Nordisk	70% NPH, 30% Regular	bacteria	U-100
Novolin 70/30	Novo Nordisk	70% NPH, 30% Regular	bacteria	U-100
Novolin 70/30 Penfill	Novo Nordisk	70% NPH, 30% Regular	bacteria	U-100
Animal insulin				
Mixtard	Novo Nordisk	70% NPH, 30% Regular	pork	U-100
Intermediate-acting				
Human insulin				
Humulin N	Lilly	NPH	bacteria	U-100
Insulatard Human NPH	Novo Nordisk	NPH	bacteria	U-100
Novolin N	Novo Nordisk	NPH	bacteria	U-100
Novolin N Penfill	Novo Nordisk	NPH	bacteria	U-100
Humulin L	Lilly	Lente	bacteria	U-100
Novolin L	Novo Nordisk	Lente	bacteria	U-100
Animal insulin				
Iletin II NPH	Lilly	NPH	beef/pork	U-100
Insulatard Human NPH	Novo Nordisk	NPH	pork	U-100
Purified Pork N	Novo Nordisk	NPH	pork	U-100
Iletin I NPH	Lilly	NPH	beef/pork	U-100
NPH	Novo Nordisk	NPH	beef	U-100
Iletin II Lente	Lilly	Lente	beef	U-100
Purified Pork Lente	Novo Nordisk	Lente	pork	U-100
Iletin I Lente	Lilly	Lente	beef/pork	U-100
Lente	Novo Nordisk	Lente	beef	U-100
Long-acting				
Human insulin				
Humulin U	Lilly	Ultralente	bacteria	U-100
Animal insulin				
Iletin I Ultralente	Lilly	Ultralente	beef/pork	U-100
Ultralente	Novo Nordisk	Ultralente	beef	U-100

SOURCE: Reprinted with permission from *Diabetes Forecast*, October 1992, p. 39. Copyright © 1992 by American Diabetes Association, Inc.

enough insulin, it's important not to dispense too much. That will cause your blood sugar to fall too low.

Most diabetics inject insulin through disposable plastic syringes and needles. Your doctor will show you how to cleanse your skin and prepare the insulin (some insulins settle at the bottom of the glass vial and need to be gently shaken or rolled between your palms to get an even suspension). You will be shown how to give yourself an injection. If you are ever unsure about this procedure, you will find step-by-step instructions on a package insert that comes with the insulin.

Patients rarely relish the thought of needles, but most find insulin injections easy to get used to. Modern ultrafine needles on disposable syringes are a blessing. Many patients find that the "stick" of these thin needles is barely noticeable.

SIDE EFFECTS   Insulin causes few serious side effects. One such side effect that is fortunately rare is a generalized allergic reaction. This can happen if you are allergic to pork or beef. The symptoms are a rash over your entire body, with shortness of breath or wheezing, a drop in blood pressure, rapid pulse, or sweating. If you experience any of these symptoms, contact a doctor immediately. Once the reaction is under control, your doctor can switch you to another type of insulin to avoid a repeat.

Diabetics sometimes encounter a second type of allergic reaction. This one occurs at the site of the injection. The skin swells and itches, and becomes reddened. The reaction lasts from a few days to a few weeks before it gradually disappears by itself. If this happens to you, tell your doctor. He or she may give you a skin test to make sure you can safely tolerate other forms of insulin. Beef insulin generally causes allergic reactions more often than pork insulin, and human insulin causes the least allergic reactions of all.

Practical Tips

- Refrigerate any insulin you are not using in a given day. Keep at room temperature enough insulin for one day; injections are less painful that way.

- All insulin will last for three years when kept cold (but don't freeze it). At room temperature, Regular insulin lasts for eighteen months and NPH and all Lente preparations last for twenty-four months. Don't use a bottle of insulin after the expiration date stamped on the label.

- If you plan to travel across more than two time zones, check with your doctor first. She or he will show you how to adjust your insulin doses to avoid swings in blood sugar levels. Take along enough insulin for the trip, plus enough portable snacks (dried fruit, nuts, crackers, hard candy, etc.) to sustain you if you miss a connection or your bus or plane is delayed.

WHAT INSULIN CAN AND CANNOT DO   Before insulin was discovered, Type 1 diabetics usually died within two years of diagnosis. Today, diabetics diagnosed in childhood or as teenagers can look forward to decades of life. Clearly, insulin is a powerful drug that can cause miraculous transformations. But every medicine has strengths and limitations. It's important for everyone who takes insulin to understand what insulin therapy can and cannot do.

For example, as long as you eat a proper diet, insulin does a very good job of keeping blood sugar under control. Thus insulin helps your body avoid the high sugar levels that all too often lead to atherosclerosis, kidney damage, and the many other dangerous side effects of diabetes. Insulin cannot control these side effects indefinitely in every diabetic. Twenty or thirty years after the onset of diabetes—sometimes earlier, sometimes later—complications can begin to set in. How closely you care for your health has much to do with when, if ever, these complications appear.

You might wonder why insulin isn't an all-perfect solution for a disease that is caused, after all, by too little insulin. One of the major reasons has to do with how insulin is delivered. People whose metabolisms function normally regulate their blood glucose levels extremely well. An intricate system of hormonal triggers keeps blood sugar within a certain range, and the moment blood sugar rises a bit too high or dips a bit too low, the body automatically compensates by sending glucose to or from the bloodstream.

The most sophisticated human inventions can only approximate this finely tuned system. Whereas the insulin delivery system in nondiabetics operates with pinpoint accuracy, continuously supplying as much or as little insulin that the body needs, insulin injections in diabetics typically deliver fixed doses of the hormone one or two times a day. The difference, explains Professor George Cahill of

Harvard Medical School, is like a refrigerator with a faulty thermostat. Instead of running only when the temperature rises, the refrigerator runs and shuts off arbitrarily regardless of whether the food is too hot or too cold. Eventually, the food suffers.

When diabetics carefully monitor their blood sugar and use a combination of diet, exercise, and medication to keep blood sugar levels in a healthy range, they keep their ailing "thermostat" in as

INSULIN INJECTION GOES HIGH-TECH ▰▰▰▰▰▰▰▰▰▰

In the beginning, there was the needle and syringe. Diabetics would use them to draw a certain amount of insulin from a glass vial, then inject the insulin into a patch of skin. This is how most diabetics still get their insulin. It's simple and inexpensive.

Then came the pump. In the early 1980s, researchers developed a battery-powered, belt-worn pump that dispensed a continuous dose of insulin, with adjustments for meals, through a tiny needle that slipped under a diabetic's skin. With its knobs and switches, it was more complicated. And it was expensive—up to $2,000 to buy and maintain one in the first year, then $300 to $500 a year thereafter. One recent innovation is a pump that can be fully implanted under the skin. Shaped like a hockey puck, the pump can hold a three-month supply of insulin, which is released through a radio transmitter controlled by the patient. The inventor, Dr. Christopher Saudek of the Johns Hopkins University in Baltimore, admits that with an estimated price tag of $10,000 to $12,000—well beyond the means of most African-Americans—the pump is a "pretty expensive hockey puck."

One of the most popular new insulin injectors is a pen-shaped device called the Novopen. The Novopen uses insulin cartridges instead of bottles, and the injection is controlled with the push of a button instead of a syringe. The Novopen is self-contained and so simple that even small children can use it with ease. "People like it because of sheer convenience," designer Bernard Sams told the *Wall Street Journal*, "and the fact that you don't look like a drug addict. Best of all is the price—about $99. The company says the cost of the pen plus insulin cartridges runs about the same as conventional needles and insulin bottles.

good a working condition as possible. But nothing can take the place of "the original equipment." As a Chicago attorney who is partially blind from diabetes told *Time* magazine, "People think you just take your insulin and you're fine." Recently, increasingly sophisticated insulin delivery systems have given diabetics better glucose control than ever before.

IF YOUR DOCTOR PRESCRIBES MEDICINE FOR HIGH BLOOD PRESSURE

Modern medicine is speeding toward new ways to help diabetics, and one of its proudest accomplishments over the years has been the development of medicine to help lower blood pressure. Hypertension, you'll remember, frequently accompanies diabetes and contributes to several of its dangerous complications.

Blood pressure medicines save lives and contribute greatly to the longevity and happiness of millions of diabetics. Like most medicines, though, antihypertensive preparations can cause side effects. These side effects are often particularly pronounced in the African-American community, because we have more severe hypertension than whites, and so we need higher doses of blood pressure medicine.

SIDE EFFECTS OF BLOOD PRESSURE DRUGS IN DIABETICS

FAMILY OF DRUGS	EXAMPLES	POSSIBLE SIDE EFFECTS
Diuretics		
Potassium-losing	Dyazide, Furosemide, Aldactazide, Enduronyl, many others	High blood cholesterol; in Type 1 diabetes, high blood sugar
Potassium-sparing	Amiloride, Spironolactone, Triamterene	Too much potassium in the blood
Alpha blockers	Prazosin	Low blood pressure when standing after sitting or lying

Continued on next page

Beta blockers	Propranolol, Metoprolol, Nadolol, Atenolol, Timolol, Pindolol	Prolonged recovery from, obscured symptoms of, and hypertension during times of low blood sugar; aggravation of blood vessel disease in extremeties; heart failure
Sympathetic inhibitors	Methyldopa, Clonidine, Reserpine, Guanethidine	Impotence; low blood pressure when standing after sitting or lying
Vasodilators	Hydralazine, Minoxidil	Aggravation of coronary heart disease; excessive hair growth
Converting enzyme inhibitor	Captopril	Kidney failure if high blood pressure is caused by narrowing of the kidney arteries

If you are taking medicine to lower your blood pressure, ask your doctor if it causes side effects, and what those side effects are (so you can be on the lookout). If you are bothered by side effects, *don't stop taking the medicine.* Instead, tell your doctor. Your doctor may be able to switch you to a medicine that's just as effective and causes fewer side effects.

Stopping medication without a doctor's consent is one of our community's most serious mistakes. It's certainly natural to want to discontinue medicine that makes us feel bad. And it may be difficult to accept the risks of heart failure, kidney failure, and even such non-life-threatening disorders as impotence and excessive hair growth from a medicine designed to help you. But these risks are much lower than the risks of untreated hypertension. So if your medicine is making you sick, speak up. Your needs are important, and they count.

Some people with diabetes have very special needs indeed. Because of their age or the demands being placed on their bodies, these diabetics deserve special consideration. Children who have diabetes pose unique challenges for their parents and other family members, as do the elderly. Pregnant women who have diabetes must manage the disease at a time of extraordinary biological and emotional stresses. In all three cases, the impact of diabetes is different among African-Americans than among whites. Let's discuss what we can do to help our most vulnerable.

HELPING OUR MOST VULNERABLE

Ask me to name a community that's hard-hit by diabetes, and I'll tell you African-Americans. Ask me to single out those groups of African-Americans whose struggle with diabetes is is more challenging than many people realize, and I'll name three: our children, our pregnant women, and our elderly.

Anyone can get diabetes. You can be as young as nineteen months, or as old as ninety-one years. You can have a white-collar job, blue-collar job, no job at all. You can be a physician, you can be a migrant worker, you can be a kindergarten teacher, you can be homeless, you can be a minister—diabetes isn't particularly choosy.

But the impact of the disease isn't distributed equally. As we see with race, diabetes comes down harder on some folks than on others, and it presents certain populations with challenges that others can scarcely imagine.

DIABETES IN CHILDREN

Think back to your childhood, if you will—a time of play and exploration, fantasy and relative freedom from the many obligations of adult life. Take your mind back to the thrill of birthday parties, the excitement of Christmas morning, the joy of your first achievements in school. And recapture the feeling of slowly mastering the world around you, the sense of empowerment and even invincibility that children feel as they step out into the world and begin to conquer it.

Now imagine an adolescent waking up one morning embarrassed at having soaked his sheets with urine during the night and suddenly out of his mind with thirst. Imagine a small girl who, late at night when her friends are dreaming of sandcastles and ponies, sits at the kitchen table anxiously devouring a massive plate of food that will do nothing to satisfy her raging appetite. And imagine a parent watching in shock as a normal, healthy child is suddenly and mysteriously overcome by vomiting and stomach pain, leg cramps, blurred vision, and fatigue, and realizing that somehow, for reasons yet unknown, the happy, carefree child they once knew is slipping through their fingertips.

Diabetes hits children like a hammer. Unlike the Type 2 form of the disease, which usually affects adults and when it does, develops gradually, Type 1 diabetes often arrives at a child's doorstep practically overnight. And when it does, the impact is enormous. Children's physical health often deteriorates so rapidly that only emergency medical care prevents them from falling into a coma. And the disease has a striking impact on emotional health as well. Once children are diagnosed with diabetes, the realization for children and parents alike that life will be different from that point on is often overwhelming. Dr. Donna Younger, director of the Youth Division at the Joslin Diabetes Center, says the emotional impact of learning that a child has diabetes is not unlike hearing that a close friend or family member has died. "The emotional sequelae [consequences] are parallel to those of the bereaved: shock, disbelief, denial, anger, and depression."

What Causes Childhood Diabetes

About 2 percent of all diabetics are under the age of seventeen. Diabetes affects roughly 115,000 American children—roughly 1 in 1,000. Why does diabetes affect one person and leave 999 untouched?

Family history plays a very direct role. If one family member has Type 1 diabetes, chances are very high that another will, too. The brothers and sisters of a diabetic child are fifteen times more likely to develop diabetes than is a sibling of a nondiabetic child. And if a child's sibling and parent both have Type 1 diabetes, the child's risk jumps to forty-five times higher than normal.

Sometimes children are the first persons in their families to have diabetes. That suggests something more than genetics is at work. Oddly enough, the other piece of the puzzle may be environmental. Back in 1985 in the United States Virgin Islands, the incidence of childhood diabetes suddenly shot up from four cases per one hundred thousand children to twenty-four cases per one hundred thousand. Then the epidemic subsided just as suddenly as it had come. "Practically every diabetes register worldwide showed an increase in the mid-1980s," University of Pittsburgh epidemiologist Dr. Ronald E. LaPorte told the *Washington Post*. "There appeared to be a pandemic—Aukland, New Zealand; Hokkaido, Japan; Finland; Poland; the Virgin Islands; Latvia; Estonia—raising the interesting possibility that something in the environment was accounting for this." For over fifty years, scientists have noticed that more cases of Type 1 diabetes appear in the winter than in the summer. Since children have more colds in the winter, researchers are zeroing in on the possibility that viruses help cause Type 1 diabetes.

Whatever the cause, childhood diabetes is rarer in blacks than in whites. We do see more cases of diabetes in black children these days than in the past. That could be because black families aren't finding it any easier to obtain health care. It could also be that the people who collect statistics on the incidence of disease are doing a better job of tallying diabetes in the black community. Overall, however, the rate of childhood diabetes in our community is low.

One reason that diabetes is rarer among black children may be that at the onset of Type 1 diabetes, black youngsters have only half as many *islet cell antibodies* than white kids do. These antibodies—proteins that activate cells that destroy foreign bodies—are a sign of immune-system activity. You may remember that one of the causes of Type 1 diabetes is an overactive immune system that starts to destroy a person's own insulin-producing islet of Langerhans cells.

When Childhood Diabetes Surfaces

Childhood diabetes is associated with periods of rapid physical growth. Black and white children alike typically develop the disease around ages ten to twelve for girls and twelve to fourteen for boys, as children begin their growth spurt in puberty. With Type 2, the signs of diabetes are gradual and may be so mild that family members may not realize they have the disease. That's one reason that about half of all cases of Type 2 diabetes go undetected. Not so with Type 1. Here the symptoms are so dramatic and swift that they're impossible to miss. After its sudden onset, the disease mysteriously subsides for a while in up to half of all Type 1 youngsters. Eventually, though, the child's pancreas loses its ability to make insulin. Within one to five years after the onset of the disease, the child is completely reliant on insulin injections.

The Prescription for Diabetic Children

Doctors give young diabetics the same prescription as they do older ones—the golden combination of diet, insulin, and exercise.

There are different schools of thought on what to feed diabetic children. Some doctors feel that youngsters should be allowed to eat whatever the rest of the family eats (except for sweets) plus snacks to prevent their blood sugar levels from falling too low. Others feel that spelling out a diet, including how much of which foods to eat, allows better control of blood sugar levels. The Joslin Center favors the latter approach. Whichever method your doctor recommends, make sure your child's diet is rich in fiber and low in fat. That will help minimize the complications of diabetes.

"Food is often a major problem for youngsters with diabetes," warn Dr. Donna Younger and colleagues at the Joslin Center. Some children—especially teenagers—overeat because of very compelling pressure to fit in with their peers, and to prove to their friends that there is nothing wrong with them. And all children go through periods of rebellion and obstinance, during which they may not be willing to stick to a prescribed diet.

Talk openly and compassionately with your child about the importance of a good diet. Young children often eat well if they are allowed to become active participants in the overall management of diabetes. So as their maturity allows, let them start testing their own blood and urine. And encourage them to express their feelings and ask questions. Diabetes invariably mystifies children, and parents who allow children to talk about the disease will relieve fears

HELPING A CHILD EXERCISE SAFELY

Strenuous exercise lowers blood sugar levels. If an exercise session is severe, a diabetic can even experience advanced signs of hypoglycemia, including loss of consciousness (passing out).

What many diabetics don't realize is how delayed the reaction can be. A recent study at the University of Wisconsin Hospital and Clinics pediatrics diabetes program showed that over a two-year period, forty-eight of three hundred young Type 1 diabetics experienced hypoglycemia anywhere from three to thirty-one hours after unusually strenuous exercise—typically running or swimming. The symptoms were most apt to appear in the middle of the night. Over half of the forty-eight youngsters developed seizures or lost consciousness.

Dr. Michael McDonald, who ran the study, says that many diabetics—and even their doctors—may not appreciate the effects of exercise on blood sugar. He calls the delayed reaction "PEP" hypoglycemia ("post-exercise and play"). "This term highlights the peppy, active patient who is likely to experience PEP hypoglycemia," McDonald told USA Today. Youngsters who are just starting exercise programs are also prone to the problem.

Exercise is very valuable for diabetics, so don't confine a child to a rocking chair for fear of hypoglycemia. Instead, take simple precautions. A child can minimize or avoid PEP hypoglycemia by eating more food before (and snacking during) exercise, and by taking less insulin that peaks during the night. It's also helpful to monitor a child's blood sugar more often on the night after vigorous exercise.

and help children develop a sense of mastery and pride about taking care of their health.

Children have different needs for insulin, depending on how old and how active they are. Most children take a combination of regular and intermediate insulin to begin with, and continue insulin even when the disease seems to lessen. When their bodies stop making insulin entirely, children must take more insulin more often. Your doctor will prescribe the proper type and dose of insulin for your child's individual needs. Children do learn to tolerate daily injections, although the development of the Novopen, which can be mastered by even a young child, has made injecting insulin much more convenient.

Unlike adults, most children get so much exercise that they don't need a formal exercise program to stay healthy. But it's important that they and the rest of the family understand how exercise affects blood glucose levels.

Caring for any child can be rewarding but difficult work. Caring for a diabetic child, even more so. In addition to putting bread on the table and maintaining a roof overhead—the normal daily concerns of all parents—parents of diabetic children must also think about timing insulin injections, planning and preparing a good diet, and numerous other measures to prevent harmful fluctuations in a child's blood sugar. African-American parents may find it particularly difficult to balance the many responsibilities of parenthood while coping with the additional demands of diabetes. In neighborhoods where a child's classmates carry guns to school, in communities where getting a job (much less keeping one) is a hit-or-miss proposition, in cities and suburbs and towns where the multiple threats of drug abuse, family violence, underemployment, and crime pull at the seams of black families, successfully managing childhood diabetes can seem next to impossible. Indeed, when researchers at Children's National Medical Center in Washington, DC, studied their records, they discovered that black children, children from one-parent households, and children without health insurance had an unusually high rate of readmittance to the hospital. The readmissions happened because of chronically high blood glucose levels caused by poor control of diabetes. Why the high

readmission rate? Low literacy, lack of information, patient manip-
ulation, family disorganization, inadequate parenting skills, and
limited money—to name just a few.

At the same time, parents and children from the most difficult
of circumstances do manage childhood diabetes successfully. It
takes a supportive family, one that works with a child compassionately but fairly. It takes parents who are wise enough to give their
child a strong sense of self and the ability to make sensible deci-
sions. It takes disciplined loved ones who are willing to embrace a
child when the child needs support, while taking care neither to be
overprotective nor to foster overdependency.

The payoff, for both child and family, is a healthy, vibrant
youngster who views care for his or her health as an important,
manageable, enjoyable part of life. I'm reminded of a story about a
well-adjusted diabetic youngster who invited her friends to see her
needles and syringes and bottles of insulin. Like Tom Sawyer, who
elevated the everyday task of fence-painting to a high privilege, she
even allowed a friend the honor of testing her urine for sugar.
These are the kinds of children I hope our community can raise.

A diabetes specialist—whether a health educator, nurse, physician, or other professional—can give you plenty of useful and reassuring advice and information about managing childhood diabetes.
You can also get information from the American Diabetes Association (see Appendix).

DIABETES IN PREGNANT WOMEN

What happens when diabetes comes face to face with one of the
strongest human instincts—the urge to bear children? Asking that
question seventy-five years ago would have brought disappointment. Back then, mothers and infants died so frequently from complications of pregnancy that young diabetics were advised not to
consider motherhood. The advent of insulin changed all that.
Today, the survival rate for infants of Joslin Clinic patients is 98
percent, and for the mothers themselves, 100 percent.

That's not to say pregnancy is a free ride. Bearing a child

always carries some risk, even when the mother is the picture of health. How does diabetes heighten that risk?

Risks to the Mother

Diabetes brings four principal risks to the mother: eye disorders, kidney ailments, nerve problems, and a disturbance in blood chemistry.

Pregnancy often worsens diabetic retinopathy to the point that women begin to lose their vision. Whereas certain retinopathies subside once a mother gives birth, others can be more permanent. If you're a diabetic and you're following the advice of the National Eye Institute by getting your eyes checked each year (are you?), then you will know how healthy your eyes are. If you have any degree of retinopathy, visit an ophthalmologist. The eye doctor will examine you and may take photographs of the back of your eye. When you visit again, these photos will serve as a baseline to let the doctor compare your eyes before and during your pregnancy.

Pregnancy doesn't cause kidney failure. But if your blood contains an unusually high amount of urea nitrogen or creatinine—two normal byproducts of protein breakdown—at the start of your pregnancy, it could be a sign of trouble. Kidneys help remove excess urea nitrogen from the bloodstream, and too much urea nitrogen in your blood could mean that your kidneys are having difficulty doing their job. To help head off the hypertension and swelling caused by too much fluid in your system, your doctor may prescribe bed rest and sometimes hospitalization.

You may feel pain, numbness, or other unusual sensations in your feet, hands, or elsewhere. This nerve disorder—neuropathy—is common and disturbing but usually not serious, and can be eased with aspirin or other pain medicine.

Diabetic women sometimes experience an accumulation of urine chemicals called ketones. These sweet-smelling substances are produced when the body breaks down fat for energy. They are a dangerous sign that tissues aren't getting glucose and the liver has run out of glycogen. Your doctor will advise you to test for ketones by periodically collecting a sample of your urine and dipping into it a chemically treated paper strip. You simply wait a few minutes and then compare the color change on the strip with a chart. One such product, Chemstrip, is available by prescription.

If you notice persistently high levels of ketones and glucose in your urine (Chemstrips measure glucose levels, too), particularly if you begin to feel nauseous or thirsty, or start to urinate a lot, call your doctor immediately. This condition can develop in less than twenty-four hours, and the effects can be tragic. While high ketone levels are unhealthy for you, they can be life-threatening to your unborn child.

Risks to the Unborn Child

Regrettably, high ketone levels aren't the only complication of diabetic pregnancies that can harm a fetus. Nearly half of the infants born at the Joslin Clinic have hypoglycemia, according to Dr. John W. Hare. And a substantial percentage have difficulty breathing, a condition known as *respiratory distress syndrome.* Stillbirths are more common among diabetic women than others, for reasons unknown. Diabetics also have a higher-than-average risk (estimated at between 4 and 12 percent) of delivering an infant with birth defects.

Reducing the Risks

For both mother and unborn child, the risks of a diabetic pregnancy can be greatly reduced by proper medical care. I'll give you an example. In 1991, two hundred diabetic women took part in a study at the University of California at San Francisco Medical School. Half of the women began treating their diabetes between six and thirty weeks into their pregnancies. The other half started aggressive diabetes treatment before conception. When the babies were delivered, twelve children born to late-starting women had birth defects. But among the women with early care, only one child had birth defects. Dr. John Kitzmiller, who organized the study, was very clear. "Our data indicate it is necessary to begin education and management before conception to prevent major congenital anomalies [birth defects] in infants of diabetic mothers."

Let me explain the elements of proper prenatal care, according to the Joslin Clinic, the respected authority on this matter. In general, remember that while pregnancy is a normal biological event, it places extreme demands on any woman's body, and even more so for a diabetic woman. Your regular routine of visiting your doctor for checkups, monitoring your blood and urine, taking your insulin, and so forth, becomes even more deliberate and careful when you carry a child. When you become pregnant, getting care from your regular physician is no longer enough. It takes a team of doctors—an internist, an obstetrician, and a pediatrician, for example. If you're lucky enough to have access to more specialized care, the ideal combination is a diabetologist (a doctor specializing in diabetes), a neonatalogist (a doctor who specializes in newborn infants), and an obstetrician.

See your doctor at the earliest possible point in your pregnancy—even before you conceive, if possible. That way, you can be referred to the proper physicians and baseline information can be gathered on your health. Sometime in your first trimester—and the earlier the better—a doctor should take your history and give you a full physical. If your eyes show evidence of retinopathy, you will be referred to an ophthalmologist. You will be given blood and urine tests.

During your first visit, you will also receive full instructions about what to expect in your pregnancy, what to watch for, and whom to contact in an emergency. Some doctors have this information available on a printed sheet, which gives patients something to refer to after the office visit. Your doctor should discuss home monitoring of your blood and urine.

One important discussion item is your diet. An unborn child requires glucose and amino acids, so you will need to eat extra carbohydrates and protein. Plan on eating an extra three hundred calories per day, less if you are overweight. Like every expectant mother, you will need more calcium to help build bones and teeth; you can get the extra calcium you need each day with a quart of lowfat milk, lowfat cheese, or calcium supplements. Multivitamins are a good idea, particularly those containing folic acid. Most pregnant women can't eat enough iron for themselves or their child, so take an iron supplement.

Pregnancy typically changes a woman's need for insulin. You may find that you need somewhat less insulin during your first trimester, and progressively more insulin as your pregnancy progresses. Most women find that their need for insulin stabilizes at the end of their pregnancy and returns to their normal level after they give birth. Your doctor will help you work out a schedule based on your individual needs.

Keeping close track of your health is so important that during your pregnancy you should see a doctor every week. During each visit, your weight and blood pressure will be recorded, your eyes will be examined, and your body will be checked for signs of swelling.

Giving Birth

Somewhere around week thirty-seven or thirty-eight of your pregnancy, you will be admitted to a hospital for delivery. You'll have some routine lab work, including blood and urine tests for glucose. A doctor will also perform an amniocentesis. The purpose of the amniocentesis is to measure certain chemicals that will tell your doctor whether your baby's lungs are mature enough to breathe on their own.

During the amniocentesis, a small amount of fluid (about four teaspoonfuls) is removed with a long slender needle from your womb. Your doctor may or may not use a local anesthetic to numb your skin beforehand. Every doctor should use an ultrasound device to locate the position of the unborn child immediately before inserting the needle. (If you walk around after the ultrasound but before the amniocentesis, the baby can shift positions.) The test usually doesn't cause complications, but the needle can sting, and you may feel cramping when it enters your womb and pressure as fluid is withdrawn.

If your baby is healthy and its lungs are strong, your doctor may decide to induce labor. This is commonly done with a medicine called Pitocin (pi-tó-sin)—also called "Pit"— which is similar to a hormone that's naturally present during labor. If your doctor wants to induce labor, ask if he or she plans to give you Pitocin. If so, ask if you can receive it intravenously. Pitosin is sometimes injected with a needle into your muscles, but it's difficult to control the dose this way. Pitocin can cause very strong contractions and potentially harmful complications for both you and your baby, so precise control of the dose is important.

If for some reason labor cannot be induced, your doctor will perform a cesarean section. Cesareans have come under intense scrutiny in recent years, partly because many cesareans—33 to 75 percent, according to the National Institutes of Health—are performed unnecessarily. But when a mother has diabetes, cesareans can be lifesavers for both mother and child.

Cesarean sections are major operations, but they are usually straightforward. Nurses shave your pubic hair and insert a catheter (a long slender plastic tube) in your urethra to collect your urine. After your abdomen is scrubbed with an antiseptic solution, you will be given anesthesia. You will have three options. Spinal anesthesia and epidural anesthesia involve injecting anesthesia with a fine needle into or near the spinal canal. The anesthesia numbs the nerves from the pelvis down through the legs and feet. With either type, you remain awake during the operation. General anesthesia, on the other hand, puts you to sleep. The anesthesia is administered either through an intravenous drip into your arm, or through inhaling a mixture of gases, or both.

Once your belly is numb, the doctor will make a horizontal incision near your pubic hair. You will feel no pain. The incision is deepened into your uterus, and the infant is gently lifted free. Many mothers find it satisfying to see their babies delivered; you can ask that drapes usually placed between you and the operating field be lowered during the delivery. Once the baby's mouth and nostrils are sucked clear of mucus and she or he is breathing well, you or your partner can hold the baby. The surgeon removes the placenta, then stitches you up.

One of the more unusual aspects about a diabetic pregnancy is that you don't have to have diabetes to experience one. Around 3 to

5 percent of healthy, normal women sometimes develop *gestational diabetes* during pregnancy. Unlike in Type 1 or Type 2 diabetes, women with gestational diabetes have plenty of insulin. The problem is that certain important hormones (including estrogen and cortisol) produced by the placenta to ensure a safe pregnancy also make the body resistant to insulin. In most mothers, the pancreas successfully compensates by simply producing extra doses of insulin. Women whose pancreas can't produce enough extra insulin to overcome the effects of the placenta's hormones develop gestational diabetes.

Gestational diabetes follows two noticeable trends. First, the condition usually starts around the twenty-fourth week and becomes more pronounced as the pregnancy progresses. That's because a growing placenta produces more and more hormones, which make it increasingly difficult for insulin to work. Second, gestational diabetes may be more common in African-American women than among white women; one Northwestern University study found that for reasons unknown, black women were nearly twice as likely as whites to develop the condition.

Since the hormones responsible for gestational diabetes are a part of pregnancy, you'd expect the diabetes to subside when a mother gives birth. This is exactly what happens; after birth, mothers with gestational diabetes return to normal. In the meantime, however, gestational diabetes presents certain risks. One of them is a condition known as *macrosomia* (from *macro*, meaning large, and *soma*, meaning body), in which the infant grows unusually large. Once insulin fails to remove enough glucose from the mother's blood, the infant's pancreas senses the high glucose levels and converts the extra sugar to fat, which is stored on the infant's body. The fat makes the baby grow bigger than usual. This can be dangerous to infants because they can be injured during delivery. Sometimes these babies are so large that they cannot be delivered vaginally, and the doctor must perform a cesarean.

Another problem is low blood sugar in the infant. This can occur when the mother has consistently high blood sugar levels, which stimulates an infant's pancreas to produce lots of insulin. Once the infant is born and the mother's high-sugar blood is no longer available, the infant's large dose of insulin quickly removes much of whatever glucose is in the infant's blood, causing low blood sugar.

And there are long-term problems as well. Children whose mothers had gestational diabetes during pregnancy can face lifelong health problems. "Our research indicates that such children can become obese, can develop diabetes themselves, and may experience abnormal intellectual growth," Dr. Norbert Freinkel, former president of the American Diabetes Association, told *USA Today*.

If you have gestational diabetes, you can minimize these complications by following the same healthful guidelines that all diabetics should embrace—eating a good diet, checking your blood for glucose and your urine for ketones, and using insulin if your doctor prescribes it. Ninety percent of the time, gestational diabetes can be cleared up through a good diet alone. If diet doesn't work, insulin is called in.

Gestational diabetes affects mothers, too. Over half of the women who experience gestational diabetes develop permanent diabetes later on. If you have gestational diabetes, your doctor should examine you periodically once you deliver. This way, if you develop full-blown diabetes, it can be caught and treated successfully at the earliest possible stages.

It's difficult to predict who will develop gestational diabetes. Doctors say you are at risk if 1) you're obese, 2) you have a family history of diabetes, 3) you have previously given birth to a large infant, or 4) your urine tests positive for glucose. But when researchers at Johns Hopkins University investigated hundreds of pregnant women who had gestational diabetes, the group with none of these four so-called risk factors was nearly as large as the high-risk group. This suggests that there are other risk factors at work besides the standard four.

One such consideration could be age; gestational diabetes may be more common in pregnant women over the age of twenty-four. But no one knows for sure what the predictors of gestational diabetes may be. So the American Diabetes Association (ADA) and the American College of Obstetricians and Gynecologists recommend that all pregnant women over the age of twenty-four be screened for gestational diabetes by taking a glucose tolerance test. (Regrettably, less than half of the doctors in an ADA survey said they usually advise their patients to get such a test.)

The reasons for screening are compelling. In the words of Dr. Norbert Freinkel, "A simple glucose tolerance test can identify 60,000 to 90,000 women who each year develop gestational diabetes." If you were one of those women, wouldn't you want to know it? Talk with your doctor about gestational diabetes. If you are a pregnant woman over age twenty-four, ask for a glucose tolerance test.

DIABETES IN ELDERS

Imagine a large room filled with one thousand African-American babies. Statistics tell us that by the time they reach age 20, 5 of them will have diabetes. By age 40, the number will climb to 25. By age 60, 125 will have diabetes; by age 70, 245.

Diabetes is like arthritis: some people have it as youngsters, but it's much more common as people age. We find that trend in both whites and blacks in the United States. But there's a racial gap in the number of Americans with diabetes, and the divide only widens as people grow older. As children, teens, and young adults, whites and blacks have the same rate of diagnosed diabetes— around 1 percent, according to the National Institutes of Health. By age forty, African-Americans have a little more diabetes—3 percent, versus 2 percent for whites. By fifty, diabetes is fully twice as common in blacks than in whites—8 percent versus 4 percent.

Then something interesting happens. With black men, diabetes rates level off. But for black women, they soar. Fifteen percent of all black women over the age of fifty-four have been diagnosed as having diabetes, compared to 9 percent of black men and 7 percent of white men and women. And that doesn't include the many blacks who have diabetes and don't know it.

Precisely why diabetes becomes more common with older age is one of the many mysteries of the disease. One reason seems to be that obesity is more common in old age. Older people also get less exercise. Advancing years also decrease the number and sensitivity of insulin receptors in the body's cells. Older people have more hardening of the arteries, which probably contributes to the wasting away of pancreatic tissue. Finally, our kidneys don't filter as well when we grow old, a trend that's particularly noticeable in blacks. Without an efficient filtration system, impurities remain in our bloodstream instead of being flushed out. That can contribute to certain forms of hypertension that are associated with insulin resistance.

I'm often struck by how fatalistically many of my elderly patients and their families view diabetes. Many assume that diabetes in old age is as inevitable as wrinkles. And most who get diabetes assume there's little they can do about it. Well, diabetes isn't inevitable in older people (it's more like dentures than wrinkles; some people get them, some don't), and when it comes, it isn't a death sentence. It's simply a health condition that people must learn to respect. If you respect diabetes and you're willing to spend a little energy on behalf of your health, your body will love you for it.

What to do is no great secret. Enjoy a sound diet, one that provides a minimum of simple carbohydrates and fat, moderate amounts of protein, and lots of fiber-rich whole grains and vegetables. Leafy green vegetables are great for older people, because they provide fiber, vitamins and minerals, and satisfying fullness. Many people are troubled with gas as they grow older. Sometimes that's because loose-fitting dentures or the lack of teeth make chewing difficult, and you swallow more air with each mouthful. But it's often because of a lack of certain enzymes in your digestive tract. One such enzyme is lactase, which breaks down the sugar (lactose) in milk, cheese, ice cream, and other dairy products. Lactase deficiency is relatively common in African-Americans, and more so with older age. Reducing dairy products in your diet or using a commercial lactase supplement such as Lactaid or Lactase can help.

Check your blood sugar frequently and take your diabetes pills or insulin as your doctor recommends. Most older people can control their diabetes with a good diet alone, particularly if they lose weight in the process.

And you're never too old to exercise. "The small amount of

available data indicate that women and the elderly can respond at least as well as younger men to exercise programs," advises Dr. Neil Ruderman of the Boston University Medical Center. Brisk walking is a terrific exercise for young and old alike. If you lead an active life, you may be able to enjoy swimming, golf, tennis, and any number of vigorous sports. Many older people enjoy dancing, bowling, and less strenuous activities. And "almost everyone, even if confined indoors, can find some form of exercise for arm and leg muscles," suggests Dr. Alexander Marble of the Joslin Center.

Review Chapters 6, 7, and 8 for a general idea of how to go about incorporating diet, exercise, and medicine into your daily life. For specifics, check with your doctor. She or he can tailor a program to your individual needs.

NEW HOPE FOR BETTER LIVES

What would happen if we found a cure for the nation's leading killer diseases? Contrary to what you may think, it wouldn't add that many years to the average American's life. So says Dr. S. Jay Olshansky of the University of Chicago, who found that curing even diabetes, heart disease, and cancer—three of the nation's biggest killers—would extend the typical American's life by only a handful of years. "Once you go beyond the age of 85, people die from multiple-organ failure," Dr. Olshansky told the *Washington Post*. Basically, they die of old age. And there's no cure for that." Dr. Olshansky urges researchers to stop trying to figure out how to extend people's lives. Instead, he suggests, try to improve the quality of life. "My God, we're already living long enough. Let's make life worth living."

As an African-American physician, I take that advice with a grain of salt. Curing diabetes may add only a few years to the "average" American's life, but let's not forget that black Americans' lifespans are five to seven years shorter than white lifespans. A medical breakthrough that amounts to only a small benefit for a privileged majority may be a godsend for an underprivileged minority.

At the same time, we need to improve the quality of our lives just like everyone else. So if you asked me to decide between enhancing black Americans' quantity of life and quality of life, I'd tell you that's really no choice at all. We need both.

In both of these tasks, science is lending a huge hand. The medical profession has come light-years in its quest to understand diabetes and to help diabetics live long and rewarding lives. Not too long ago, it was impossible for many diabetics to buy life insurance without paying exorbitant rates. Today, diabetics can obtain life insurance at near-normal premiums. "They [insurance companies] can see the improvement," wrote Jack Apfel as vice chairman of the International Diabetes Federation. "Today we, the diabetic community, feel more in control and know we can have a normal life. We can fit diabetes into our lives and not fit our lives into the diabetes."

NEW WAYS OF PREVENTING DIABETES

Type 1 Diabetes

A generation ago, doctors were relatively helpless against Type 1 diabetes, multiple sclerosis, lupus, and thirty-five other autoimmune diseases—diseases in which the body's sentinels somehow attack the tissues they are supposed to protect. "There was no way to think about treating these diseases—absolutely none," immunologist Dr. Malcolm Gefter of MIT told the *New York Times*. Today, the tangled mystery of autoimmune diseases is unraveling. In the words of Dr. Hugh McDevitt of the Stanford University School of Medicine, "We're within a gnat's hair of understanding everything we need to know about how the immune system reacts."

These advances are allowing unprecedented therapies designed to prevent Type 1 diabetes. In the mid-1980s, researchers in Canada and Europe gave newly diagnosed Type 1 diabetics an immunosuppressive drug called cyclosporin. The hope was that this would halt the immune system's destruction of insulin-producing beta cells in the pancreas. The drug worked so well that after one year, 25 percent of the patients didn't have to take insulin.

Hope rose that if persons susceptible to Type 1 diabetes could be located, the disease could be blocked before it took hold.

But cyclosporine caused serious side effects. And like a broad-spectrum pesticide that injures more than the garden pest it is intended for, cyclosporine wasn't very precise. One scientist compared cyclosporin therapy to "hitting a bull's-eye with a bazooka." And so the search was on for a medicine as effective as cyclosporin but without the side effects.

A few years later, paydirt. At the University of South Florida Health Science Center, researchers gave daily doses of a drug called Imuran to fourteen-year-old Peggy Polopolus. Polopolus's sister, grandfather, and two aunts had diabetes, and doctors predicted the teenager would develop the disease herself within six months. Five years later, Polopolus had no diabetes—and no side effects. The news was so exciting that normally cautious scientists let their hair down a bit. "This is an extraordinarily promising avenue for study," one expert at the National Institute of Diabetes and Digestive and Kidney Diseases told the *Los Angeles Times*. "I don't want to overstate its significance, but this could really be hot stuff." Work is now underway to test Imuran in eighteen thousand persons across the country who have a sibling, child, or parent with diabetes.

In the late 1980s, researchers at the same University of South Florida Health Science Center scored another breakthrough in the push to prevent Type 1 diabetes. They wondered if the benefits of immunosuppressive therapy weren't caused so much by the immune-suppressing drugs, but by large doses of insulin that were given along with them to fight the drugs' tendency to raise blood sugar. They tried giving newly diagnosed Type 1 diabetics two-week megadoses of insulin. What they found was intriguing. During their two-week reprieve, the pancreatic beta cells went into hibernation, producing only one seventh the usual amount of insulin. But once the beta cells had been granted a temporary vacation from their insulin-producing duties, they went on to pump out insulin with renewed vigor. Even after an entire year, these pancreas glands produced twice as much insulin as those of other newly diagnosed diabetics who were treated with conventional doses of insulin to keep blood sugar low.

The researchers reasoned that the body's autoimmune response is somehow activated by too much beta cell activity. And if you can give beta cells a rest early on, you can prevent the onset of diabetes. "If we treat prediabetic high-risk individuals and if we can stop the progression," one scientist told *Science News*, "then they may never have to take [daily] insulin. That's what we'd like to achieve."

Of course, the first step to treating high-risk persons is figuring out who is at risk. And on that front, researchers got a major boost with the discovery that diabetes is preceded by the destruction of a protein in the pancreas. The protein, called 64K because of its large size, is destroyed by certain antibodies (proteins that attack foreign matter). And those antibodies are present as long as seven years before the start of diabetes. Find those antibodies, American Diabetes Association medical director Dr. Mark Kahn told the *Los Angeles Times*, "and it's a virtual certainty that person will develop diabetes within three years." Work is now proceeding to reduce the cost of screening for 64K antibodies from $500 to about $2, which would make the test commercially viable.

Some prevention research is focused on heading off the complications of Type 1 diabetes. Once someone has diabetes, the fine blood vessels in their eyes and kidneys are at risk. Stanford University researchers have found a blood protein whose presence becomes measurably conspicuous as early as eighteen months before any blood vessel damage occurs in the eyes or kidneys. Measuring bloodstream levels of the protein, called prorenin, may one day save diabetics from blindness or kidney disease by warning doctors to start aggressive treatment early.

Type 2 Diabetes

With Type 2 diabetes, prevention is proving a more difficult nut to crack. Still, though, there are breakthroughs. For example, we may be able to predict Type 2 diabetics twenty or thirty years before the disease breaks out. In southern Arizona, scientists have discovered that healthy, nondiabetic youngsters from the Pima tribe have an average of 15 to 20 percent more insulin in their bloodstreams than do healthy nondiabetic white youths. This is a sign that the body responds sluggishly to insulin. And insulin resistance is known to lead to diabetes. If we test high-risk persons early in life and find higher-than-normal insulin levels, we may be able to prevent the onset of Type 2 diabetes by starting them on a good diet and stressing weight control.

The mineral chromium may play a role in preventing Type 2 diabetes. A high-chromium diet seems to enhance the body's ability to transport glucose from the bloodstream to the body's cells. In tests sponsored by the United States Department of Agriculture's Human Nutrition Research Center, researchers gave chromium supplements to eight men and women whose glucose intolerance signaled they were prediabetic. After receiving chromium supplements for about a month, the volunteers were given a glucose tolerance test. In seven of the eight persons, blood sugar levels rose nearly 50 percent less than before the chromium supplements. The amount of chromium the volunteers received—two hundred micrograms—is within the government's recommended daily allowance for the mineral (fifty to two hundred micrograms). But chromium-rich foods are scarce. The easiest way to boost your chromium level is to limit your intake of simple sugars, which rob your body of chromium.

NEW WAYS OF TREATING DIABETES

Monitoring Blood Glucose

Imagine being able to monitor your blood sugar without drawing blood. If David L. Purdy has his way, it won't be too long before bloodless glucose monitoring makes fingerpricks obsolete. Purdy's company, Biocontrol Technologies, Inc., of Indiana, Pennsylvania, is developing a device that shines a beam of harmless infrared light at a patient's skin. "The light will measure the blood through the skin tissue," Purdy explained for the *Indiana Gazette*. The skin reflects some of the light back to a sensor in the device, which detects the amount of glucose in the blood. A digital display shows the glucose reading. The device is presently in the testing stages.

And in San Francisco, a University of California professor has come up with an idea for using a skin patch to measure bloodstream glucose levels. While using patches to deliver medicines to the skin, Dr. Richard Guy noticed that other chemicals were coming out of the skin. Guy hit on the idea of using patches to help measure blood glucose levels. Tests with mice have already shown that the amount of glucose that winds up on the patch correlates nicely with the amount circulating in the animal's bloodstream. The professor is working with Cygnus Therapeutic Systems of Redwood City, California, to develop a skin sensor for diabetics. "Ideally, we'd like something like a dot on the end of an eraser," the firm's research director told *Scientific American.* "But we can certainly go for a patch or cuff."

Delivering Insulin

Have you ever wondered why insulin must be injected? The reason is that your stomach and intestines would digest the hormone before it could act, so an insulin pill would be worthless.

But there are other ways to deliver medicines into the bloodstream. Human skin is being tested as a potential delivery system for insulin. In Massachusetts, researchers at Harvard Medical School and the Whitehead Institute for Biomedical Research are transferring insulin-producing genes into skin grafts. Their hope is that a diabetic's skin could one day produce insulin just as easily as a normal pancreas does.

Some of the more dramatic new developments in insulin delivery go straight to the heart of the problem: the impaired pancreas itself. In severe cases of diabetes, when a patient is slipping away fast because of complications, surgeons can now transplant a human pancreas. This eliminates the need for insulin injections, while stopping the progression of kidney disease and nerve disorders. Patients who receive a new pancreas must forever take immunosuppressant medication, lest the body attack the new pancreas as alien tissue. Thus the surgery is usually performed for patients who are getting a new kidney and therefore will need to take immune-suppressing drugs anyway.

These medicines can be risky, notably because suppressing the immune system makes people prone to infection. Could there be a way to boost a person's insulin production without relying on immunosuppressives? For years, researchers have wondered if diabetes could be treated by providing an insulin-deficient person with a fresh supply of pancreatic beta cells. One of the chief roadblocks was thwarting the body's immune system, which would normally destroy foreign beta cells just like it would a virus or germs.

But in 1991 researchers at the Washington University School of Medicine in St. Louis found an ingenious solution. Dr. Paul Lacy placed beta cells into thin tubes that were then implanted under the skin of laboratory mice. The tubes, made of a special porous membrane, allowed oxygen and other nutrients to nourish the pancreatic cells, while preventing entry of immune-system attack cells, which were too large to fit through the pores in the membrane. The tubes worked. Soon the pancreas cells were responding just like a healthy pancreas, producing insulin when blood sugar levels rose, and cutting back when they fell. Eighty percent of the diabetic mice who received the tubes became healthy within sixty days. When the implants were removed, the mice became diabetic again. If tests on larger animals show the same encouraging results, Dr. Lacy hopes to try the tubes on human volunteers by 1994.

Ultimately, Dr. Lacy and other researchers working to develop membrane-protected beta cells are striving to create an artificial pancreas, one that would provide diabetics with natural, effective blood glucose control without the need for daily injections. Once human tests are completed in the mid-1990s, we could be one step closer to automatic blood glucose control.

A MULTIPRONGED APPROACH
FOR GOOD HEALTH

There is no shortage of research ideas as we push toward the day when diabetes is cured. If the past provides an example, we may be in for a few surprises. Scientists have already found a virus (of all things) that can prevent diabetes in mice. And in Boston, researchers have stumbled across a naturally occurring hormone called insulinotropin, which may control blood sugar levels in Type 2 diabetes better than insulin does. Research labs throughout the world are addressing the prevention and treatment of diabetes from a number of angles, and exciting breakthroughs in the coming years are inevitable.

But for this research to have the most relevance to African-Americans, it must target our needs. The federal government funds $130 million in diabetes research each year, dispensing research grants to universities and hospitals throughout the country. Although diabetes has reached epidemic proportions in minority communities, only 15 percent of those tax dollars go to study diabetes in minorities, according to a 1992 study by the United States General Accounting Office. "The magnitude and effects of diabetes in black Americans remain relatively unstudied," concurs a 1990 report by the National Institutes of Health, "despite evidence that [Type 2 diabetes] is more prevalent and conveys more extensive morbidity [disease] in this group than in the general population."

At the same time, it will take more than appropriately directed research to end the diabetes crisis in the black community. The health care system must change as well. Doctors must be educated to the special risks of diabetes in the African-American community, and they must respond with swiftness. Too many physicians simply don't understand the circumstances that make diabetes among African-Americans a killer disease. And when diabetes takes its toll, too many experts blame the victims instead of reforming a health care system that's frequently inaccessible, unaffordable, and unreliable. "The obligation calls on the health care system to figure out how to work with people who have different perspectives, not to get people to accommodate to how we've designed the system," Dr. Howard Spivak, Massachusetts deputy commissioner of public health, explained to the *Boston Globe.* "We've got to move, not them."

Finally, even after the nation achieves health care reform, we African-Americans will still be obligated to do our part. We must respect our bodies. We must eat soundly. We must keep our weight under control. We must develop a habit for enthusiastic exercise. We must get the best medical care that we can, and we must then take our doctor's advice seriously. Despite America's dazzling technological accomplishments, despite the headlines that spill out of our nation's labs, the bottom line for millions of black Americans will remain what it has been since the first African-American came down with diabetes: we must practice disciplined, careful self-care.

Look at it as a point of pride. Imagine your ancestors gazing upon you as you care for your health, and smiling. Because they know you are guaranteeing your best possible chance for a long and rewarding life.

RESOURCES

To get more information about diabetes, call or write to the organizations listed below.

GENERAL INFORMATION

The American Diabetes Association (ADA) provides booklets and information on free educational and screening programs held each November (National Diabetes Month). You can get a free one-year subscription (four issues) to ADA's colorful newsletter, *Diabetes*, on request. For $24 you can become a member of ADA and receive twelve monthly issues of *Diabetes Forecast* magazine. ADA also sells cookbooks (including holiday cookbooks), children's books about diabetes, and menu plans.

American Diabetes Association
1660 Duke Street
Alexandria, VA 22314
(800) 232-3472

The National Diabetes Information Clearinghouse, a branch of the National Institutes of Health, can send you free educational materials, including nutrition information, a diabetes dictionary, a fact sheet on diabetes in African-Americans, and a directory of local diabetes-related programs for black Americans.

National Diabetes Information Clearinghouse
Box NDIC
Bethesda, MD 20892
(301) 468-2162

For free information about federally sponsored research on diabetes, contact:

National Institute of Diabetes and Digestive
and Kidney Diseases
National Institutes of Health
Building 31, Room 9A04
Bethesda, MD 20892
(301) 496-3583

The American Society of Diabetes Educators trains and certifies physicians, registered nurses, occupational therapists, registered pharmacists, and other health professionals in diabetes care and provides educational materials for professionals. The Society can refer you to the certified diabetes educator nearest you.

American Society of Diabetes Educators
500 North Michigan Avenue
Chicago, IL 60611
(800) 338-3633

DENTAL COMPLICATIONS

The National Institute of Dental Research can mail you a free pamphlet on diabetes and periodontal disease, plus information on ongoing research.

National Institute of Dental Research
National Institutes of Health
Building 31, Room 2C35
Bethesda, MD 20892
(301) 496-4000

DIABETES IN CHILDREN

The Juvenile Diabetes Research Foundation has educational pamphlets and emergency cards for children.

Juvenile Diabetes Research Foundation International
432 Park Avenue South
New York, NY 10016
(800) 223-1138

EYE COMPLICATIONS

The National Eye Institute provides free educational material for people who may be at risk of diabetic eye disease, or for people who have been recently diagnosed as having glaucoma or diabetic retinopathy. The Institute can also refer you to other organizations and give information on ongoing research.

National Eye Institute
National Institutes of Health
Building 31, Room 6A32
Bethesda, MD 20892
(301) 496-5248

KIDNEY DISORDERS

[See "General Information"]

PAYING FOR DIABETES CARE

The government provides free medical care to many thousands of black diabetics through Medicaid (which provides coverage to the poor) and Medicare (which covers presons over sixty-five and those with certain disabilities). With Medicaid, the federal government requires states to provide certain services (for example, inpatient and outpatient hospitalization, laboratory testing, physician services, and others). States are also required to provide care to all Medicaid-eligible persons under twenty-one years of age. Other services are optional. For instance, not every state pays for podiatrists' services for diabetics who need foot care. From state to state, Medicaid eligibility guidelines and the range of available services vary greatly. To learn who is eligible for Medicaid in your state and what services are provided, phone your state Medicaid agency or local department of social services.

Like Medicaid, Medicare pays for medical services deemed reasonable and necessary for the treatment of diabetes and other illnesses. The program pays for physicians' services, diagnostic testing, and a range of other services. Medicaid pays for certain medicines, but it does not pay for self-administered medicine, like insulin (see below for how to obtain free insulin and other self-administered medicines). For information on Medicaid benefits in your state, call your local Social Security office or department of social services.

Many large drug companies have programs to help low-income patients obtain medicines free of charge. Companies generally provide this service to patients who are not eligible for private or public health insurance, but there are exceptions. Your doctor must contact the company on your behalf.

Insulin

Have your doctor contact:
Indigent Patient Program Administrator
Eli Lilly and Company
Lilly Corporate Center
Drop Code 1844
Indianapolis, IN 46285
(317) 276-2950
(317) 276-9288 (FAX)

Blood Pressure Medicine

For information on antihypertension drugs made by **Lederle Laboratories**, ask your doctor to contact a local sales representative for the company. For the name of the sales representative nearest you, your doctor can phone the company at (914) 735-2815 from 8:00 a.m. to 4:30 p.m. EST.

Boehringer Ingelheim Pharmaceuticals, makers of Catapres and other blood pressure medicines, will send your doctor an application form explaining the company's guidelines. The doctor can determine whether you are eligible based on the guidelines. The doctor must submit an application form and a prescription each time he or she makes a request. The company says "recommendation by a social worker is beneficial." Your doctor should contact:
Mary Eisenmenger
Partners in Health Program
Boehringer Ingelheim Pharmaceuticals, Inc.

900 Ridgebury Road
PO Box 368
Ridgefield, CT 06877-0368
(203) 798-4153

Bristol-Myers Squibb Company, makers of over a dozen heart medicines, offers free medicine to patients 1) whose doctors are enrolled in the company's Cardiovascular Access Program; 2) who aren't eligible for health insurance; and 3) who are financially eligible, as determined by a "means" test and a "liquid assets" test. Doctors can obtain a three-month supply of medicine. Your doctor should contact:
Bristol-Myers Squibb Cardiovascular Access Program
PO Box 9445
McLean, VA 22102-9998
(800) 736-0003
(703) 760-0049 (FAX)

CIBA-GEIGY Pharmaceuticals, makers of Apresolin, Esidrix, and other blood pressure medicines, will send eligibility guidelines to your doctor. Have your doctor contact:
Jackie Laguardia, Administrator
Patient Support Program
CIBA-GEIGY Corp.
556 Morris Avenue, D-2058
Summit, NJ 07901
(800) 257-3273
(908) 277-5849

ICI Pharmaceuticals, makers of Zestril, will supply your doctor with application forms through company headquarters or a local sales representative. The company provides automatic refills of one- to three-month supplies of medicine for up to one year, after which your doctor must reapply every twelve months. Have your doctor contact:
ICI Pharmaceuticals Group Patient Assistance Program
Yvonne Graham, Manager
Professional Services
ICI Pharmaceuticals Group
PO Box 15197
Wilmington, DE 19850-5197
(302) 886-2231

Knoll Pharmaceuticals, makers of Isoptin, operates the Heart-in-Harmony Program for patients taking Isoptin. You can receive educational information and hints on enhancing compliance with your doctor's prescription. For more information, call the company's toll-free Patient Help Line, (800) 444-0559.

For free medicine, your doctor must forward a request to a local Knoll sales representative or to:

Knoll Pharmaceuticals
30 North Jefferson Road
Whippany, NJ 07981
(800) 526-0710

Marion Merell Dow, makers of Cardizem, targets patients with incomes below the federal poverty line. In addition to providing a three-month supply of medicine at any one time, the company encourages physicians of low-income patients to provide free services. The company will send your doctor forms for you to fill out. Have your doctor contact:

Indigent Patient Program
c/o Bill Lawrence
Supervisor for Product Contributions
Marion Merrell Dow, Inc.
9300 Ward Parkway, West 2
Kansas City, MO 64114
(816) 966-4000
(816) 966-3825 (FAX)

Merck, Sharpe, & Dohme, makers of Diupres and Diuril, accepts letters from physicians of a patient's medical needs, the existence of financial hardship, and a patient's inability to qualify for private or public health insurance. Have your doctor contact:

Merck Indigent Patient Program
Professional Information Division
Merck Human Health Division—U.S.
West Point, PA 19486
(215) 540-8600

Diabetes Pills

Pfizer, Inc., manufactures Diabinese and Glucotrol, which reduce blood glucose levels. The company also makes the antihypertension medicine Procardia. Your doctor, who must waive his or her treatment fee, writes a letter to Pfizer explaining that the patient is poor and has neither private health insurance nor Medicaid, and enclosing a prescription for the product. The company will send refills if your doctor resubmits the request. Have your doctor contact:

Mr. Richard Vastola
Manager, Industry Affairs
Pfizer Indigent Patient Program
Pfizer, Inc.
235 East 42nd Street
New York, NY 10017
(212) 573-3954

If you live in Arkansas or Kentucky and live below the federal poverty line, have no health insurance benefits, and do not qualify for government entitlement programs, Pfizer will provide any of its medicines free of charge. In Arkansas, patients must be certified by a local County Department of Human Services. In Kentucky, patients must be certified by the Kentucky Cabinet for Human Resources. In both states, your doctor must waive his or fee for the initial visit; in Kentucky, the fee waiver extends to all visits. Have your doctor contact:

Ms. Pat Keller
Program Director
Arkansas Health Care Access Program
Arkansas Health Care Access Foundation
PO Box 56248
Little Rock, AR 72215
(501) 221-3033
(800) 950-8233
or
Mr. Arch Mainous, Jr.
Executive Vice President
Kentucky Health Care Access Foundation
147 Market Street, Suite 200
Lexington, KY 40507
(606) 255-7442
(606) 254-5846 (FAX)

Searle, makers of Aldactazide, Calan, and Kerlone, allows your doctor to decide if you are eligible for free medicine. The company gives eligibility guidelines, but they are not requirements. Searle will give your doctor Patient in Need Program certificates, which you take along with a prescription to any pharmacy. The pharmacy will give you the free medicine and be reimbursed by Searle. Have your doctor contact:

Administrator
Searle Patients in Need Foundation
5200 Old Orchard Road
Skokie, IL 60077
(800) 542-2526, (708) 470-6633 (FAX)
or a local Searle sales representative at (800) 542-2526.

Kidney Medicine

Amgen, Inc., makers of the kidney medicine Epogen, provides free replacement medicine to patients with annual adjusted gross family incomes of less than $25,000 and no public or private health insurance. Patients with insurance or with incomes of $25,000 to $50,000 may be eligible for free replacements after the company considers income level and out-of-pocket expenses. Any dialysis center, physician, or hospital may apply on behalf of a patient. You must reapply every twelve months. Contact the "Safety Net Program for Epogen" at the company's Medical Technology Hotline, (800) 272-9376, or (202) 637-6698 in Washington, DC.

Central Pharmaceuticals, Inc., makers of Niferex-150 capsules, has an Indigent Oral Program. Have your doctor contact:

American Kidney Fund
6110 Executive Boulevard, Suite 1010
Rockville, MD 20852
(301) 881-3052
(301) 881-0898 (FAX)

Ortho Biotech makes the anemia medicine Procrit available free of charge to patients who meet certain medical criteria and lack the money and insurance to obtain treatment. The company requires that participating physicians not charge low-income patients for their services. Your doctor can get an eligibility application form from Ortho Biotech product specialists or by contacting:

The Ortho Biotech Financial Assistance Program
1800 Robert Fulton Drive, Suite 300
Reston, VA 22091-4346
(800) 447-3437

GLOSSARY

Aerobic exercise—any exercise that stimulates the heart and lungs by involving large numbers of muscles.

Amino acid—a building block of protein.

Anaerobic exercise—exercise that increases muscle strength but doesn't give your heart and lungs a good workout.

"Apple" physique—a body shape marked by excess belly fat.

Atherosclerosis—a buildup of fatty plaque that can cause hardening and narrowing of an artery, leading to heart disease or stroke.

Autoimmune disease—an affliction in which the body attacks itself. Said of Type 1 diabetes.

Blood glucose monitor—a device that measures the amount of glucose in the blood.

Cataract—cloudy spots on the lens of the eye. It is a complication of diabetes.

Complete protein—protein from food that contains all eight essential amino acids.

Complex carbohydrate—starch or fiber.

Cortisol—a hormone manufactured in the adrenal glands that teams up with glucagon to produce glucose from body fat or muscles. It is used when the body's immediate supplies of glucose are low.

Creatinine—a byproduct of normal protein breakdown. High levels in the blood can signal kidney problems.

End-stage renal disease—irreversible kidney failure often requiring dialysis or kidney transplantation. It is often caused by diabetes.

Essential amino acid—any of the eight amino acids that we must obtain from our diet because the body does not manufacture it.

Eye pressure test—a test for glaucoma that checks for the buildup of pressure within the eye. It is not sufficient for determining whether a person has diabetic eye disease.

Fat-soluble vitamins—vitamins that can be stored in fat tissues for later use. They are vitamins A, D, E, and K.

Gestational diabetes—a form of diabetes caused by hormonal changes in pregnant women.

Glaucoma—buildup of pressure inside the eye. It is a complication of diabetes.

Glucagon—a hormone that signals the liver to break down glycogen to glucose when glucose supplies are low.

Glucose—a simple sugar that is the body's principal fuel.

Glucose tolerance test—a measure of how well a person's pancreas manufactures insulin. The patient drinks a sweet beverage and has blood drawn at intervals. It measures recent (short-term) blood sugar levels.

Glycogen—long chains of glucose molecules. It is one way the body stores excess glucose.

Glycosylated hemoglobin—a blood chemical formed when bloodstream glucose sticks to hemoglobin. It is a long-term measure of a person's blood sugar levels.

Hypertension—high blood pressure.

Hypoglycemia—low blood sugar.

Incomplete protein—protein that contains some but not all of the essential amino acids.

Insulin resistance—unresponsiveness of the body's cells to insulin.

Islets of Langerhans—small clusters of cells found throughout the pancreas. They produce insulin.

Ketones—chemicals found in urine when the body is having extreme difficulty moving glucose out of the blood.

Lente—an intermediate-acting insulin that reaches peak activity three to ten hours after injection.

Low blood sugar—insufficient glucose in the blood. It is caused by too much insulin or diabetes medicine, too little food, or exercise without food, and can cause coma or death.

Macrophage—a scavenger cell of the immune system.

Nephron—a filtering tube in the kidney. It produces urine.

Nonessential amino acid—any one of 14 amino acids that the body produces on its own and therefore does not have to be supplied through the diet.

NPH—an intermediate-acting insulin that reaches peak activity three to ten hours after injection.

Obesity—clinically, 20 percent or more over a person's ideal weight.

Pancreas—the gland responsible for insulin secretion.

"Pear" physique—a body shape marked by excess fat on the thighs and buttocks.

Pupil dilation test—a method by which an ophthalmologist determines whether a patient has diabetes-related eye disease.

Purified—an insulin that contains less than .001 percent proinsulin protein.

Regular—a fast-acting insulin that reaches peak activity in one to two hours.

Retinopathy—a condition marked by leaky capillaries and the buildup of scar tissue inside the eye. It is one of the principal complications of diabetes.

Retrograde ejaculation—leaking of semen into the bladder during ejaculation.

Semilente—a fast-acting insulin that reaches peak activity in one to two hours.

Simple carbohydrates—glucose, fructose, sucrose, lactose, or other carbohydrates made of one or two molecules of sugar. Also called simple sugars.

Standard—an insulin that contains up to .001 percent proinsulin protein.

Sulfonylureas—pancreas-stimulating pills.

T-cell—an immune-system cell that destroys viruses, debris, and other material harmful to the body.

Type 1 diabetes—diabetes marked by low or nonexistent insulin production. Also called insulin-dependent diabetes mellitus, or IDDM.

Type 2 diabetes—diabetes marked by insufficient insulin to meet the body's needs, or resistance to insulin. Also called noninsulin-dependent diabetes mellitus, or NIDDM.

Ultralente—a long-acting insulin that maintains peak activity over a 24-hour period.

Urea nitrogen—a byproduct of normal protein breakdown. High levels in the blood can signal kidney problems.

VLDL—very low density lipoprotein. A form of blood cholesterol that may contribute to the risk of heart disease and that is reduced after exercise.

NOTES

Chapter 1: What Is Diabetes?

page 1: According to the historical documents, which are known as the *Papyrus Ebers* (after Georg Ebers, who obtained them in 1872 at the site of the ancient Egyptian city of Thebes), Egyptian physicians prescribed at least four remedies for diabetes. Here is one:

Cakes	
Wheat grains	1/8
Fresh grits	1/8
Green lead earth	1/32
Water	1/3

Let stand moist; strain it; take it for four days.

page 11: Throughout the world, Type 2 diabetes isn't always caused by excess body weight. In Ethiopia, where Type 2 diabetes is the predominant form of the disease, diabetics are of normal weight. But in America, Type 2 diabetes and obesity are very strongly linked.

Chapter 2: What Does Diabetes Do?

page 16: Narrowing of blood vessels occurs mostly in medium-sized vessels called arterioles. The blockage is caused not only by a physical obstruction (the clot) but also by muscle spasms. That's why vasodilators (medicines that relax the blood vessel wall) reduce a person's blood pressure, often within a matter of seconds.

page 18: In addition, blindness from diabetic retinopathy is three times more prevalent in black women than in black men.

page 23: The likelihood of white women receiving a kidney was 12 percent lower than for white men, but still placed white women ahead of black men and black women.

Chapter 3: Black Folks at Risk

page 32: The death rates among whites increased over this period, too, but not as much as the black death rates. In 1920 about 60 out of every 100,000 elderly whites died of diabetes. Whites died from diabetes about twice as often as blacks. By 1970, the black death rate had surpassed that of whites, which stood at about 160 deaths per 100,000 persons.·

page 35: Another explanation for high diabetes rates in black women is that black women may produce and use insulin differently than others. Researchers who have studied the residents of Bogalusa, Louisiana, in a long-running heart study say that black children, especially black girls, produced more insulin than white children did. Black children were also unusually resistant to insulin. Both conditions can set up a black youngster for developing diabetes later in life.

Chapter 4: So You've Got "Sugar"

page 47: Sometimes blood samples are also tested for something called *glycosylated hemoglobin.* When a molecule of glucose in the bloodstream comes in contact with a molecule of hemoglobin, an iron-rich blood pigment, the two stick together like Velcro®. The higher your blood sugar has been, the more glycosylated hemoglobin a scientist will find in a blood test. "When blood sugar rises above a certain level, it irreversibly attaches to hemoglobin, and that glycosylated hemoglobin persists for the life of the red blood cell—about 120 days," Dr. James R. Gavin III of the University of Oklahoma Health Sciences Center explained to *McCall's.* This is a good way to measure your average blood sugar levels over a period of weeks. In contrast, the glucose tolerance test measures short-term blood sugar levels (over a period of hours).

Ketones are poisonous pleasant-smelling compounds (the acetone in fingernail polish remover is a ketone) that are produced by the breakdown of fat when the body can't use glucose in the blood and has exhausted its supply of glycogen (stored glucose) in the liver. Their presence in the urine suggests that the body is having extreme difficulty moving glucose out of the bloodstream.

page 47: The amount of glucose consumed in the glucose tolerance test is less for children. The blood glucose level numbers refer to milligrams of glucose in a deciliter of blood, or mg/dl.

page 47: Doctors say a person has a condition known as impaired glucose tolerance if the blood glucose level is under 140 at the start of the glucose tolerance test, over 200 during the test, and between 140 and 199 two hours later. Impaired glucose tolerance is a condition between normal metabolism and full-blown diabetes.

page 55: The *Journal of the National Medical Association* is not to be confused with the *Journal of the American Medical Association.* The National Medical Association is a professional organization of black physicians dedicated to serving the black community. It was formed in 1895 in response to the American Medical Association's refusal to admit black physicians. This position was AMA's official policy from the 1870s until the late 1960s, when the Association was forced to respond to the civil rights movement that was sweeping the country.

Chapter 5: Living with Diabetes

page 61: People with diabetes are still instructed to monitor their urine for ketones, particularly during illness, pregnancy, and other stresses.

page 69: The general rule about stress raising blood sugar levels holds true for Type 2 diabetes. For Type 1 diabetes, findings are more mixed. Some studies show that stress raises blood sugar levels; others that stress lowers them.

page 71: The National Survey of Black Americans also found that black Americans with the highest levels of psychiatric disorders were likely to suffer other serious health problems, such as ulcers, hypertension, kidney disorders, and cardiovascular problems.

Chapter 6: Watching What You Eat

page 79: One study that caused scientists to rethink the role of sugar happened at the

University of Minnesota, where researchers fed five kinds of breakfasts to twelve Type 1 diabetics, ten Type 2 diabetics, and ten nondiabetics. All meals had similar types of total nutrients, but each meal had a different kind of carbohydrate. Some contained a potato, others a pancake, others refined fructose (fruit sugar), sucrose (table sugar), or glucose. People have always assumed that sugars produce a much higher rise in blood sugar than complex carbohydrates (starches). But after the meal, people who ate the glucose breakfast had the largest rise in blood sugar, and the fructose breakfast gave the smallest increase. The sucrose, potato, and pancake breakfasts all tied for second. As one researcher told *Science News*, "While sucrose is not better than complex carbohydrates, it's not worse either."

page 81: A gram is a very small unit of weight. A saltine cracker weighs about one gram.

page 84: In some diabetics, a diet high in complex carbohydrates increases the level of bloodstream fats known as *triglycerides.* This increase will show in a blood test, so be sure to tell your doctor that you are trying to achieve better blood glucose control by increasing your intake of complex carbohydrates.

You may find that certain fiber-rich dried beans and vegetables (kidney beans, pinto beans, cabbage, broccoli, and many others) cause gas, which can be uncomfortable and embarrassing. Cutting down on the offending foods can help. You may also find useful a liquid enzyme preparation called Beano®, which when added to food helps reduce the amount of gassiness and bloating in your abdomen. Beano® is available in supermarkets and natural food stores.

page 104: If you lose more weight than one or two pounds per week, the excess weight loss is *not* fat.You're either draining water from your body, or even worse, burning your muscles for calories. Either way, you're hurting yourself. Protect your body by striving for gentle weight loss at all times.

Chapter 7: Exercising Your Options

page 107: A man who weighs 165 pounds will burn about 500 calories in an hour by bicycling at 10 miles per hour or swimming with light to moderately hard strokes.

The discussion of exercise pertains to Type 2 diabetes, the form of diabetes that has been included most often in exercise studies.

page 108: One simple exercise that's recommended for bedridden patients is to lie for a minute or two with your legs elevated at a thirty to sixty degree angle. Then sit up and dangle your legs over the side of the bed for a few minutes before lying on your back again for five minutes. You repeat the cycle three to six times in a session, three or four times a day. This routine, called *Buerger exercises,* is not known to increase glucose management. But the mild exercise is great for improving blood flow to your legs and feet and for helping to keep your muscles toned and strong, according to the Joslin Clinic. It also helps relieve the boredom of an extended hospital stay.

page 109: In a blood pressure reading, the higher number (*systolic* pressure) indicates blood pressure when the heart pumps. The lower number (*diastolic* pressure) indicates blood pressure when the heart rests.

page 110: People who are fat run a higher risk of cancers of the colon and rectum, along with cancers of the reproductive organs (breast, uterus, ovaries, cervix, and endometrium in women; prostate in men).

Chapter 8: Taking Your Medicine

page 121: An Indonesian scientist even found that a diet of green beans and onions lowers blood sugar.

page 124: If the price of insulin is beyond your reach, most major drug companies have programs to provide medicine free of charge to patients who would otherwise not be able to obtain them. See Appendix for details.

Chapter 9: Helping Our Most Vulnerable

page 141: In fact, researchers can tell pretty much who will develop childhood diabetes by measuring a person's antibody levels and measuring their insulin levels. A child in a prediabetic state would produce lots of antibodies and little insulin. Looking at the presence of diabetes in the child's family would provide further confirmation. Scientists hope to use these tests to give families advance notice that a child is likely to develop diabetes, thus helping families to avoid the crisis that can occur when a child begins to show undiagnosed diabetes symptoms.

page 142: Of course, the risk of diabetes in a family with a history of diabetes increases regardless of whether family members know they have the disease. A child whose parents developed Type 2 diabetes before middle age stand an 80 percent chance of developing diabetes themselves.

INDEX

177

ABOUT THE AUTHORS

WALTER LESTER HENRY, JR., M.D., M.A.C.P., has over fifty years experience treating and researching African-American diabetics and is the author of numerous scientific papers on metabolic disorders. He is affiliated with many organizations, including the American College of Physicians and the American Board of Internal Medicine.

KIRK A. JOHNSON is editor of the *Journal of Health Care for the Poor and Underserved*, published by Meharry Medical College in Nashville, TN. He has taught journalism and public policy at Tufts University and testified before Congress on health protection for minorities. His writing appears in national publications such as *Essence*.

MAUDENE NELSON, M.S., R.D., a registered dietitian and certified diabetes educator, is a staff associate at the Institute of Human Nutrition, College of Physicians & Surgeons, Columbia University, and a nutritionist for the Arteriosclerosis Research Center at Columbia-Presbyterian Medical Center.

LINDA VILLAROSA is a senior editor at *Essence* magazine, specializing in medical and health topics. She has also written for *American Health, Mademoiselle, Ms., the New York Times Book Review*, and other national publications. Her articles have received numerous awards and honors.